CONQUER YOUR CHRONIC PAIN

CONQUER YOUR CHRONIC PAIN

A Life-Changing Drug-Free Approach
for Relief, Recovery, *and* Restoration

PETER ABACI, MD

New Page Books
A Division of
The Career Press, Inc.
Wayne, NJ

CONQUER YOUR CHRONIC PAIN
EDITED BY PATRICIA KOT
TYPESET BY PERFECTYPE, NASHVILLE, TENN.
Printed in the U.S.A.

To order this title, please call toll-free 1-800-CAREER-1 (NJ and Canada: 201-848-0310) to order using VISA or MasterCard, or for further information on books from Career Press.

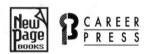

The Career Press, Inc.
12 Parish Drive
Wayne, NJ 07470
www.careerpress.com
www.newpagebooks.com

Library of Congress Cataloging-in-Publication Data

CIP Data Available Upon Request.

For my father, Zeki.

ACKNOWLEDGMENTS

I have been blessed over the years to work with so many compassionate and innovative clinicians at the Bay Area Pain & Wellness Center. Your hard work and huge hearts are a constant inspiration. For most of my career, I have had the good fortune of working side by side with Dr. John Massey, who has a heart of gold and a never-ending passion to heal. Special thanks go to Michael Sullivan, Christine Hirabayashi, Rachel Votaw, Lucrecia Martinez, and Karlee Holden for your valuable ideas and insights.

I am also indebted to the thousands of patients who have invited me into their lives and bestowed their trust upon me. In particular, I would like to recognize Eric Morton and Brandon Anderton for opening up and sharing your brave stories to our readers.

Gratitude also goes out to my agent, Andrea Hurst, for always believing in me and my mission; Barry Fox for your patience with my creative process; Lauren Manoy, Adam Schwartz, Laurie Kelly-Pye, and the rest of the team at Career Press/New Page Books; and to Justin Loeber and the team at Mouth Public Relations.

Lastly, a big hug to my wife, Pamela, and our kids, Anthony and Gabriella, for being so understanding and supportive throughout the whole process.

CONTENTS

Introduction: What Makes the Doctor Feel Good.............11

Chapter One: The Politics of Pain........................19

Chapter Two: The "Pain Brain"..........................37

Chapter Three: The Abaci Plan...........................51

Chapter Four: Find Calm in the Storm.....................61

Chapter Five: Reframe Harmful Thoughts..................83

Chapter Six: Ignite Creativity........................... 99

Chapter Seven: Use the Medicine of Movement.............111

Chapter Eight: Ingest Quality............................127

Chapter Nine: Recharge.................................145

Chapter Ten: Gain Treatment Perspective 155

Chapter Eleven: It's Just a Matter of Time.................167

Afterword: Two Steps Forward, One Step Back.............179

Notes...185

Index...189

About the Author 192

What Makes the Doctor Feel Good

Can you imagine being able to walk into a room and have the power to do something that will make somebody's pain go away?

Being able to change the way a person feels for the better, and in just a matter of minutes, is an exhilarating feeling for a doctor. A patient comes to you with debilitating pain in his or her back, leg, or neck, and you have the ability to perform a procedure or deliver a medication that quickly dissipates that person's pain. Back when I was starting off as a doctor in training, that was my idea of a rush. What a major league baseball player feels after hitting a game-winning home run, or a concert pianist after opening night, that was what I felt after treating a patient's pain.

While in medical school at the University of Southern California (USC), I became good friends with a bright, happy-go-lucky class-mate named Jack. During downtime from class, we often played pick-up basketball games with the guys, went to Trojan football games on weekends, lifted weights together, and mostly kept each other laughing through the stress of medical school. Back then I was unde-cided about which field of medicine I wanted to go into, but Jack was sure he wanted to become an anesthesiologist. He seemed to know quite a bit about the specialty, perhaps because his mom worked as an administrator in the anesthesia department at USC. Jack eventually convinced me that a career in anesthesia would be challenging, rewarding, and at the same time, would mean I would only have to deal with any given patient's complex medical problems for a finite period of time. The opposite would be true in a career based on chronic disease management. Anesthesia seemed like a great choice.

Jack and I stayed at USC for our anesthesia residencies, which meant we spent a lot of time working and training at Los Angeles County Hospital, one of the largest and busiest hospitals in the country; in many ways, a world unto itself. A major trauma center serving vast numbers of indigent patients from the greater Los Angeles area and beyond, County Hospital was loaded with people suffering from every conceivable disease, including some not usually seen in the United States. Crises were as routine as your morning cup of coffee. Every minute of every day, people with gunshot wounds, stab wounds, fractured skulls, and limbs torn off in motorcycle accidents were rolled or dragged in through the hospital doors. On many Saturday nights, we worked frantically to save people who had been caught up in what we referred to as the "knife and gun club." People were born in that hospital, died there, and those without homes sometimes even lived there.

It was exciting to have patients' lives literally in my hands all day long, and I soon became determined to make sure that each and every one of them woke up pain-free. The more cases I handled, the better I got at titrating medications so that patients would wake up feeling very comfortable, no matter what type of surgery they had undergone. And by the time I reached my senior year of residency, I very much wanted to apply my pain-relieving skills outside of the operating room. As it happened, there was a brand new specialty associated with anesthesia that dealt with pain management, so that became my senior elective.

During this rotation, I was introduced to painful diseases like diabetic neuropathy, trigeminal neuralgia, complex regional pain syndrome, and herniated discs. I learned how to relieve these terrible, long-standing pain problems by performing special nerve blocks and other high-tech procedures. The results were instantaneous and made me feel great. Let's face it, being able to walk into a room and do something on the spot that wipes away someone's pain gives you a god-like feeling! And using cutting-edge technology that few other doctors have mastered made me feel even more special. So once my anesthesia residency was complete, I went to the University of California at San Francisco for a fellowship in pain management.

There, my program director introduced us to a new concept: How about considering the patient as a *whole,* rather than focusing exclusively on the area where the pain seemed to be originating? This philosophy of medicine, called the *biopsychosocial* model, is based on the premise that emotions, thoughts, and cultural biases all play integral roles in a person's disease and his or her ability to function in society. And in order to treat a patient effectively, all of these issues must be addressed. For chronic pain, this means understanding how a person's pain influences her emotional state and ability to get through the day, work and interact with others, and more. Then these issues can be addressed as part of a larger problem that *includes* but is not limited to the pain.

While the biopsychosocial model had been around for decades, during my fellowship the idea of applying it to the treatment of pain was still novel. And there were problems, which still remain today. Academic training centers are notorious for neglecting to provide long-term patient follow-up. Fellows are very busy mastering high-tech procedures and spinal implants, and the proper use of designer medications, so they don't have much time to think about their patients' health and well-being over the long term. And even if a fellow does happen to be curious about the long-term effects of the medicines, procedures, and surgeries, she may only see a given patient for a few weeks or months before she moves on or the patient does. So if a fellow prescribes a new medication or injection today, he will never really know how it might affect that patient a year or two down the road. As a result, doctors in pain management are not trained to think in terms of long-term outcomes or the big picture. And neither was I.

Shortly after my training was completed in 1996, I opened a pain management practice. My new practice offered patients the most up-do-date medicines, injections, and procedures, as well as special spinal implants. Since I was the new, young "whiz kid" with a fellowship in a brand-new specialty, other doctors sent me patients with complex pain problems that they couldn't solve. These doctors evidently expected me to pull some sort of rabbit out of a hat that could eliminate the pain—and the patients were desperate for me to do so. I would have liked to apply the biopsychosocial model that made so much sense in school, but it didn't seem to exist in the real world. Typically, the patients weren't receptive to it. "I have real pain; I'm not crazy," they would say. The other doctors didn't support it because my approach was nontraditional, and the insurance companies usually refused to cover my comprehensive approach. Nobody wanted a new model of healthcare; they just wanted me to do something to fix the problem as quickly as possible. In short, the biopsychosocial model had strong support in the halls of academia, but it didn't seem to be feasible in everyday practice.

Practice What You Preach

It wasn't just my observations of patients whom we failed to help that gave me pause. I was also struggling through my own experience with pain. I had long been an enthusiastic athlete, suffering the usual injuries. In my late twenties, I tore the ACL (anterior cruciate ligament) in my right knee while playing soccer. Luckily, with the help of surgery and rehabilitation, I recovered. But a few years later, after completing my medical training, I tore just about every ligament in the same knee while playing basketball. This time I didn't bounce right back after surgery, and the pain refused to go away. Medications were of little help and left me feeling sick to my stomach. I couldn't get a good night's sleep because every time I turned over in bed, the pain woke me up.

But since I was self-employed, I felt I had to return to work immediately; my family, employees, and patients were depending on me. I'd struggle through the day on crutches that made my armpits perpetually sore, ignoring the knee pain, and returning home at night with a very swollen right leg. Just getting around was a problem; I felt trapped in my own body. Soon, I realized I was forgetting things. A patient, a nurse, or my wife would tell me something, and fifteen minutes later I would forget it. Due to the ongoing pain, difficulty sleeping and getting around, plus constipation and other side effects of the medicine I was taking, I soon became depressed. And hearing about other people's pain, or watching the news and seeing the terrible things that were happening around the world, just seemed to increase my own pain.

I was going through what many of the patients had complained to me about: Above and beyond the pain, which was bad enough, I was suffering from forgetfulness, trouble focusing, depression, pain in other parts of my body, and medication side effects. I was putting on weight and my cholesterol went through the roof. I began to despair, fearing that I would never recover; my life was coming apart. In the past, I had always listened sympathetically to my patients, but I didn't understand what it was like to be in their shoes. Now it was happening to me; my pain was taking over my own life. I thought, "There must be a way to work myself out of this!" And there was. My pain led me on a journey that turned out to be my greatest medical learning experience.

At that time, articles in the medical journals focused on managing pain *symptoms,* and researchers looked for new medications and pathways that could better manage these symptoms. But neither the articles nor the researchers offered any recipes for bettering the *lives* of the patients sitting in front of me in my office.

Realizing that chronic pain patients deserved a more effective path, my new practice partner, John Massey, MD, and I began developing a comprehensive approach to helping patients recover from challenging life situations like major back surgery. We had seen that many of the medications we'd been relying on could be more of a problem than a solution, so we were no longer content to use them, alone, to manage a patient's pain. In fact, we'd seen that many of the people who took the most medicine still suffered from the greatest amounts of pain. We wanted to help people manage their pain more effectively, which would likely mean they would be taking less medication.

For example, when we saw a patient with chronic back pain who had been confined to a wheelchair for five years, we thought about ways of getting him out of the wheelchair and helping him overcome his fear of the pain, so he could lead an independent life. Rather than acting as symptom managers and adjusting his medication dosage with each visit, we began to address lifestyle changes and other comprehensive approaches that could help him get better.

We then started telling all of our patients we wanted to give them tools that would help them manage their pain more successfully, function better, and lead better-quality lives—tools that would help them sustain these improvements over the long run, as well.

After speaking with local doctors, physical therapists, and other healers, we put together a program that included physical exercises, meditation, art therapy, nutrition, tai chi, help with detox, and much more. Each patient was educated about pain in general, as well as his or her condition, and given a structure to use in building a specialized lifelong program. Because each person's pain problem was unique, we adapted the training to his or her specific needs and provided a wide array of tools and techniques. For example, one person with back problems can't bend over and tie his own shoes, while another with a painful shoulder can't reach overhead to blow dry her hair. The same conceptual approach will benefit both patients, but each needs unique therapies and exercises to overcome specific deficits. It's quite a challenge to treat a condition like chronic pain, which has 100 million different versions, using methods that can be reproducible and reliably effective!

It was difficult to convince our patients, their doctors, and the insurance companies to cooperate, but after a few years, people started to take note of the success stories coming from our clinic. We eventually discovered that the patients who took the least amount of medicine, or none at all, did better, improved their functioning in daily life more, and were more likely to return to work than those who took the strongest pain killers. They were more self-empowered to manage their pain and less dependent on doctors like me. They were also more likely to see improvements in their personal relationships.

But there was still resistance to the idea that a "whole person approach," geared to helping people become more active, healthy, and wellness-focused, works the best in overcoming chronic pain. Luckily, science-based outcome studies, along with our own data, continued to support what we were trying to do. In 2006, a study published in the *Journal of Pain* demonstrated that comprehensive pain programs such as ours "offer the most efficacious and cost-effective, evidence-based treatment for persons with chronic pain."[1]

Packaging the "Secret Sauce"

Within a few years of implementing our new approach, Dr. Massey and I saw tremendous results. Our patients were getting off their medications and improving the quality of their lives. Other doctors began calling us, asking if they could come study our methods, as did some insurance companies and healthcare investors. More importantly, we saw patient after patient creating happy endings to their stories. Many overcame their pain, and many more were able to reclaim their lives.

Yet, if there is so much evidence showing that an integrated approach to chronic pain is much more successful than the standard approach—including that presented in the *Journal of Pain* study— why are so many Americans still suffering? The reason is simple: There are powerful forces supporting the use of treatments that not only don't work, but stand in the way of those that do work. Pharmaceutical companies, medical device manufacturers, insurance companies, national policymakers, and others, including some patients, are pushing hard to keep this failed system in place, an issue I'll explore in chapters to come.

In the meantime, it's important to understand that while we all want a "magic bullet" to wipe away our pain, it won't take the form of a medicine or some new kind of surgery. Instead, the true "magic bullet" is the understanding that chronic pain is a brain-based disease, and that relief will only come from working to heal this "pain brain." Only when the brain is physically restructured and restored to health can the process of pain relief take place. This may be the opposite of what doctors have been telling people for decades, but it is backed by the latest science emerging from the lab. The true "magic bullet" for chronic pain is the understanding that both the problem and the cure lie within.

CHAPTER ONE

The Politics of Pain

Start by doing what's necessary, then what's possible,
and suddenly you are doing the impossible.
—St. Francis of Assisi

Speaking with 32-year-old Heather was a draining experience. As a newly minted pain specialist, I had been asked to assess her head, neck, and shoulder pain, which had been plaguing her since she slammed into a wooden fence while chasing down a fly ball during a softball game. I actually had to read that part of her patient record a couple of times, for it was very hard to believe that this tired-looking woman slumped in a chair could have been dashing around a softball diamond just one year earlier. Now, simply walking was nearly impossible for her, for with every step, severe pain shot from her shoulders to the top of her head.

Depressed and anxious, unable to participate in any of her favorite activities—even going out for coffee with friends had become too difficult—Heather went from being an athlete to being "a champion sitter," as she put it, who had packed on thirty pounds in just twelve months.

According to her chart, Heather was on a number of different medications, but she still suffered from debilitating pain, plus depression, and had trouble doing her usual chores. The pain made sleeping through the night very difficult, no matter how many pillows she piled up, or how many different mattresses or sleeping aids she tried.

"I'm desperate to get a good night's sleep," Heather told me, "but either I'm awake because of the pain, or I have nightmares about hitting my head that keep waking me up." Constantly fatigued, Heather had trouble concentrating at work and was terrified of being fired from her job as a bookkeeper.

"My boss stuck me in the back room," she told me, her tone tinged with embarrassment. "I think it's because no one likes to see me grimacing and fidgeting all day as I try to get comfortable. Some of my work has been given to other employees because it takes me so much longer to get things done these days. And I can't even do what's left; at least, not very well. I have to write down every single thing because I'm so forgetful. Sometimes I even forget that I made a note. I can't remember when I'm supposed to pick up the kids, when their events are coming up at school, or what they told me ten minutes ago." She added, ruefully, "I'm not much of a mother anymore."

Since her injury, Heather had seen her primary care physician many times. He did his best to help her by trying various medications, then referring her to a bevy of specialists, including two neurologists, two spine surgeons, a psychiatrist, a pain specialist, and numerous physical therapists.

"But nothing has helped much," she sighed. "And a lot of them look at me *that way*."

"Which way is that?" I asked.

"Like I'm faking it because I'm really a drug addict who wants more drugs, or I'm some kind of nut. But I'm not a nut and I'm not a fake!" she said indignantly, her eyes tearing up. "Why won't someone believe me?! I'm not making this up!"

Then she handed me a picture of a beautiful young woman with a big smile and shining eyes, standing next to a handsome young man. They had two smiling little children in their arms. I almost gasped out loud at the difference between the picture and the woman sitting before me.

"This is the *real* me," she insisted. "That's my husband and kids. We look like a happy family, don't we? And we were, but now I snap at the kids when they ask me for something. I really feel guilty about that—and about not wanting to be intimate with my husband anymore. I mean, I *want* to; I love him, and he's so nice to me. But when I come home I just . . . I don't know, I just avoid everyone, go into the bedroom, close the door, and watch TV. I don't even like to be touched anymore; I'm afraid it will make me hurt worse. But that's not me! I don't like the way I behave now, and I don't like the way I look with all this weight. I just don't like me anymore."

How could the medical system have failed her so miserably?!?

A Daunting Problem

When I began practicing pain medicine in the 1990s, spinal surgery was really taking off. Armed with new diagnostic tools, implantable devices and surgical techniques, surgeons often operated on patients who had very complicated problems: long-standing chronic pain, associated difficulties such as depression or anxiety, addiction to pain medicines or other substances, work injuries, economic hardship caused by an inability to work, and more. Surprisingly, all of these problems were addressed anatomically. That is, the doctors used MRIs and other diagnostic tools to find some physical anomaly in the body that might be causing the problem—like a bulging disc—then tried to fix it. It's kind of like examining a person suffering from diabetes, finding elevated blood sugar, treating it with insulin, and believing you've cured the disease. Yet all you've really done is brought the blood sugar level down to normal temporarily; the underlying disease process continues.

Unfortunately, with this approach, most chronic pain patients left the hospital with *more* pain and *greater* anxiety, taking *stronger* medicines, and finding themselves *less* able to return to work or re-engage in other meaningful life activities. I often saw patients for the first time at this point, after they had been thoroughly disappointed by standard medical care. Why did standard treatment fail so often? Because chronic pain is not just a "body problem" triggered by a bulging disc, hairline fracture, strained muscle, or some other physical malady that refuses to heal. *Chronic pain is an interconnected body–brain problem.* It starts with a body issue, but soon causes physical changes to the brain that quite literally turn a healthy brain into a "pain brain." Just like an errant immune system that attacks the body in the form of rheumatoid arthritis or lupus, the "pain brain" perversely floods the body with pain signals. And while the pain itself is bad enough, over time it leads to additional problems, including depression, forgetfulness, anxiety, fear, problems with work and relationships, and much more. Think of the "pain brain" as the accumulation of all of the changes that have taken place within your central nervous system that perpetuate your pain experience. It is the remodeling of the brain into an irritated, sensitive, inflamed, and beaten-down version of itself that must be overcome so that you can successfully conquer your chronic pain. We will dive deep into the latest science discoveries about the "pain brain" in the next chapter.

In the early days of my practice, I did what everyone expected of me, managing pain with the latest medications and procedures. But after I had seen many patients over the course of years, it became clear to me that while standard treatments could often reduce pain over the short run, they were not very good at decreasing it over the long haul, or eliminating it entirely. They were "quick fixes," not lasting solutions. Dismayed, I began delving into the scientific literature, "studying the studies" as it were. And two things quickly became apparent.

First, the overwhelming majority of studies on pain patients were flawed because they didn't follow the patients for a sufficient length of time. They showed good results over the course of days, weeks, or several months, but they didn't look at what happened after many months or years.

Second, even a casual look at the "pain numbers" made it clear that the health system was failing its pain patients. The numbers were frightening back then and today they're even worse. In 2011, the Institute of Medicine, which is part of the National Academies of Sciences, Engineering, and Medicine, reported that:

- At least 100 million American adults (one-third of the U.S. population) suffer from chronic pain—more than the combined total of people suffering from cancer, heart disease, and diabetes.

- Chronic pain costs the nation between $560 billion and $635 billion *every single year* to cover the costs of medical treatment and lost productivity. (This does not factor in the cost of human suffering, which is incalculable.)
- Caring for chronic pain patients places an enormous strain on the nation's medical resources, taking time and resources away from the treatment of other ailments.

When one-third of the population continues to suffer from the same disease, there is clearly a problem with the treatment being offered. More than that, as you will see, the entire system for dealing with chronic pain is seriously flawed. Despite more and more powerful drugs and cutting-edge diagnostic tools, flashy high-tech procedures and surgeries, and huge amounts of money spent on the problem, more people are suffering from more serious chronic pain than ever before. And the problem is only growing worse.

That's why the authors of the Institute of Medicine study called for a "cultural transformation in the way pain is viewed and treated." Unfortunately, they did not offer a blueprint for that transformation. While everyone seems to agree that the problem is daunting, finding the best approach is a difficult task. We now know that medicating patients heavily isn't the answer. Yet the primary focus of pain therapy continues to be how best to distribute pain medications. This is not acceptable! It is time we offer chronic pain sufferers paths to true and meaningful change. Medicine must stop being part of the problem and become part of the solution. For a major transformation to take place, chronic pain treatment must stop revolving around unnecessary surgeries and how many pills to give or take away. We must develop a deeper understanding of pain, the true goals of treatment, and ways to promote sustainable recovery.

Kate's Story

Forty-seven-year-old Kate went to see her primary care physician, complaining of low back pain.

"It's been hurting for months," she explained. "I'm not sure what caused it; it was just there one day and kept getting worse."

"On a scale of 1 to 10, how would you rate it today?" the doctor asked.

"Six," she replied. "But it's not just the pain. I'm having trouble getting around, so I have to rely on my husband and daughter a lot. And it's hard to sit all day at work."

After examining her and looking through her previous medical records for any clue to the cause of the pain, the doctor ordered an X-ray and gave the Kate a referral to physical therapy, plus a prescription for an NSAID—a more powerful version of a popular pain pill available over the counter at drug stores.

Physical therapy went well, with Kate's pain rating dropping to a 4 while she was undergoing therapeutic massage and TENS. But shortly after the therapy ended, her pain began to increase, so she returned to her primary care physician.

"It's now a 5 or a 6," she replied, in answer to his question about her pain level.

"I'm sorry the physical therapy didn't do the trick," he said. "Your X-ray showed a little disc degeneration, but nothing that would explain this level of pain. Tell you what. I'm going to give you a prescription for some stronger pain medicine. An opioid. It should do the trick. I'm also going to send you to an orthopedist to take a closer look at your back."

Kate was relieved. Surely the stronger medicine would control her pain and the specialist would figure out what was wrong—then fix it!

The orthopedist performed his own examination of Kate, asking her questions, asking her to bend this way and that to see what triggered the pain, and more. Concerned, he ordered an MRI of her back, which showed degenerative disc disease and a bulging disc.

"It's not huge," he said as he pointed to an area on the MRI. "But you can see the bulge right here. And see how the spaces between these discs are narrow compared to the other discs? That's degenerative disc disease. There's inflammation in the area, and that causes pain. It's what we call the 'pain generator.' I'm going to refer you to an interventional pain specialist, an expert in dealing with problems like this."

A few weeks later, Kate was lying on a table in an outpatient surgery center as the interventional pain specialist injected anti-inflammatory medication into her back. Working carefully, guided by a type of live X-ray called fluoroscopy, he injected the medicine in exactly the right spot.

"I'm glad we caught this when we did," the pain specialist said, smiling. "You should be fine."

Kate was indeed fine for a few days, but then the pain returned. Over the course of several months, she returned to the pain specialist several times, and each time he injected medicine into her back. Unfortunately, her pain grew more intense, not less.

"I can't believe it got worse!" she said to her primary care physician. "It's a 7 now, sometimes an 8, especially after I've been sitting all day at work. It's hard to sleep; I have to take a pill every night. I don't clean the house or shop anymore; my husband and daughter have to do all my chores. Isn't there something else you can do?"

"Well," the doctor replied, "I can send you to a different pain specialist. Maybe he'll find something the first one missed."

The second pain specialist agreed that the problem was the disc bulge and spinal degeneration, and injected a different medication into Kate's back. But like the other medicines, it only helped for a while before wearing off. Meanwhile, the pain remained severe and Kate became depressed. She couldn't get through the day without popping pain pills and antidepressants, and wouldn't even think of trying to sleep without taking sleeping pills. The pain and depression kept her from doing anything other than dragging herself to and from work: no more visits with friends or relatives, no more brisk morning walks in the park, no more nights out with the girls.

A year after that first visit to her primary care physician, Kate was a wreck. She was in constant pain, depressed, withdrawn, and feeling guilty about "turning my back on my family." Not only that, she had packed on 25 pounds and developed hypertension (elevated blood pressure). Her primary care physician put her on antihypertensive medicines and admonished her to eat better and exercise.

"Oh, great," Kate sighed to her husband. "Another thing to feel guilty about."

Desperately hoping to find relief, Kate saw a neurosurgeon referred by her primary care physician, and agreed to have spinal fusion surgery. Although the surgery seemed to go well, it took her an awfully long time to recover. Twelve months after the surgery, she was still taking large doses of opioid pain killers, as well as antidepressants and medicines for anxiety and sleep. Because she wasn't able to return to work following the surgery, and her health insurance didn't cover all of her costs, the family budget was seriously strained. Family relations were also pushed to the breaking point.

"I don't know when my husband and I last had sex," Kate sighed. "I'd like to, but . . . and there's *another* thing to feel guilty about."

"My recliner chair is pretty much my life," she continued. "I sleep there because it hurts too much to lie flat. And since I'm not at work, I sit there all day watching TV; my daughter even brings me my meals there. I used to try to keep up with my friends through Facebook, but I gave it up. Seeing what they're doing just makes me cry. The surgeon said he wanted to put a spinal cord stimulator in my back. I said okay because I want this to end, but I really don't have much hope."

Is Your Doctor Set Up to Fail You?

Kate's story is sad but not unusual. You may have gone through something similar yourself. But let's think it through again from a doctor's point of view to understand why we can't simply tweak the system a little bit to solve the problem of chronic pain.

As a whole, we doctors are well-trained and dedicated to making you well. That's what drives us: We love to heal! What we didn't realize back in medical school is that there are many pressures on physicians that make it difficult to stay focused on the patient's best interests. No matter how hard we try, we cannot dodge these pressures, because we're forced to work within a broken system. And the dysfunction is present at many levels. To begin with, the system rarely covers the type of integrated care needed to treat pain adequately, which usually means doctors are not allowed to provide the best treatment for chronic pain. As a result, we struggle every day to work with patients who have very challenging pain problems, but do not have the best tools at our disposal. In addition, the pressure to see patients quickly and do something *now*, pushes us to prescribe medicines and order tests, rather than dig deep into what's happening with our patients. Our current healthcare system, then, presents doctors with a multifactorial dilemma. Let's take a look at some of the key problems and pressures.

There are time pressures. While most doctors would prefer to spend as much time as necessary with each patient, and then spend more time thinking about the situation and perhaps discussing it with colleagues, they can't. With the costs of running a medical practice spiraling upward, while reimbursements from insurance companies and the government shrink, doctors are forced to see too many patients per day. I could write a whole book on the subject, but let me simply point out that Medicare (the federal government's program for senior citizens) pays the primary care doctor about $70 for a follow-up visit. Ideally, the doctor and patient should have a lengthy conversation during follow-up visits, with the patient describing how he has fared, how and why his pain has gotten better or worse, how it has affected his ability to get through the day, whether his emotional state has been worsened, how the various medicines are working, and more. Then, the doctor would spend time educating the patient about things like the "pain brain" and lifestyle changes, while working through a plan. But how often does that really happen? It's simply not cost-effective.

Think back to Kate's case: Her primary care physician didn't look into her lifestyle or personal history, ask how her work ergonomics might be causing or contributing to her pain, or ask whether or not she was under stress. He went straight to tests and medicines, and when the X-rays showed an anomaly in her back, passed her on to the next doctor. That's not unusual, for there is minimal reimbursement for educating patients about things like spinal anatomy, lifestyle changes, work ergonomics, controlling stress, or reframing how they look at their pain. It can take many hours—hours doctors don't have—to educate patients about stretches, exercises for the back, breathing exercises, lifestyle coaching, and so on. But the system simply doesn't support it. This means the doctor is forced to become a *symptom manager* rather than a healer and educator, prescribing medicines for pain, sleep, depression, and more, hoping that it will all somehow work out.

Even doctors who work for large groups—the current trend in healthcare—are under pressure to see more patients each day. These salaried doctors are encouraged to meet quotas and are chastised if they don't see enough patients. There is no focus on the quality of the time spent with patients. But such "assembly line medicine" is not very effective when treating complex chronic problems and diseases.

The bottom line is that the system for treating pain doesn't work well because the insurance model doesn't work well. More Americans suffer from chronic pain than from heart disease, cancer, and diabetes combined, yet our insurance system is set up to treat those diseases, not pain. Clearly, the system needs to be changed so doctors can provide better treatment, more meaningful change, and better outcomes for pain patients.

And even if a doctor does somehow manage to find the time necessary to educate patients, he or she is still pressured to prescribe medicines for pain, sleep, depression, and other problems, or to offer injections, because that's what most patients want. Seized by pain, their relationships falling apart, finances shredded, and entire lives running down the drain, people want instant results. And they've been told, over and over again by pharmaceutical company advertisements, that relief is spelled "m-e-d-i-c-a-t-i-o-n." Many medicines are advertised on TV, radio, in popular magazines and on the Internet—it seems as if people are exposed to more advertising about treatment on the Internet than anywhere else. Concerned spouses, family members, or friends who are caring for the patient also push for more medications. (I recently had a spouse come to my clinic with his intimidating two dogs in tow to make sure I understood that his wife needed stronger pain killers to get through the week!) This means that doctors, even those who would rather try different approaches, are under tremendous pressure from multiple sources to offer pain medicines.

Naturally, doctors want to be nice and give people what they want; that's human nature. But many of them also prescribe out of fear of the surveys patients fill out to rate their satisfaction. In the not-too-distant past, dissatisfied patients could not do much except vent their unhappy feelings about a doctor to family and friends. That might cost the doctor a patient or two, but no more. Today, unhappy patients can post negative remarks and ratings on various websites and, if the doctor works for a healthcare company, give an unsatisfactory rating on a customer satisfaction survey. Too many unsatisfactory ratings may cost the doctor her job, so she's under a lot of pressure to keep her patients happy, even if it means writing prescriptions she believes are not necessary—or even harmful, if the patient misuses them.

This same pressure from patients often pushes doctors to order MRIs and other tests they may think are unnecessary. Every patient that comes to my office seems to have an MRI or want one. It's as if you're not American unless you've had an MRI. You would think that the more tests the better, but if you perform enough of them you'll eventually find something "wrong," some anomaly that doctors and patients can seize upon. Then they say, "Ah ha! This is it!" and focus all of their attention on it. Unfortunately, the anomaly doesn't explain the whole pain picture. It can even turn into a red herring that diverts attention from real problems like neuroplastic changes in the brain.

The truth is, most doctors don't approach chronic pain as a brain/body phenomenon. General practitioners and primary care physicians learn little to nothing about pain management in medical school. Most doctors get zero training in managing pain unless they take a pain fellowship. So they rely on the information they get from the pharmaceutical or surgical hardware sales representatives who visit their offices, sponsor educational presentations, and charm them at medical conferences, where fancy booths filled with slick displays and brochures trumpet the benefits of their products. Sometimes the border between physician education and salesmanship is very gray. And let's face it, there are no companies peddling products to doctors that make pain patients healthier; there is no financial incentive to do so. It's all about managing symptoms, trying to fix something that's anatomically wrong, or treating the side effects of medications.

Even pain specialists can be misled. They may read the latest articles published in pain medicine journals, but most of this material covers basic science and does not offer practical guidance for day-to-day practice. This means that even pain specialists get most of their practical information about pills, injections, implants, and surgeries at sponsored events and medical conventions, where they are inundated with information presented by the firms that make the medicines and the spinal fusion hardware. Although the speakers at these conferences are experts in the field, there is an excellent chance they are being sponsored by (and therefore influenced by) a Wall Street–driven pharmaceutical or medical technology company with a large wallet.

A diligent doctor might try to dig out the latest information on his own by searching the scientific literature, but she would run into the problem of "disappearing studies." Many studies are sponsored by pharmaceutical or bioengineering companies. A fair number of these studies are never published or discussed at medical conventions, quite possibly because their results indicate that the medicine or spinal fusion hardware is either not useful or not safe. If the results are not what they hoped for, these companies simply act as if these studies never existed, and most doctors don't know the difference. Thus, a doctor searching through the medical literature might see lots of positive studies about a certain medication or type of spinal fusion hardware, but no negative studies, because those have been "buried."

Surprisingly, even insurance companies pressure doctors to prescribe pills and injections—not directly, but indirectly—by making doctors jump through a lot of hoops to get approval for other forms of treatment, like the comprehensive pain-control program we run at my center. Programs like these are not covered by most private insurance companies or by Medicare.

This makes it very difficult to get approval from an insurance company for anything other than standard treatments like medicines, tests, injections, implants, surgeries, and physical therapy. The doctor who wants to do something different must write a letter to the company, call various people, send in copies of reports, answer objections, and more. All of this is incredibly time-consuming and frustrating. Some doctors will jump through one hoop after another, determined to offer the best-possible care to their patients. But others are not so resolute. And often, no matter how much of a fight you put up, the insurance company will simply say "no," and that's it. Insurance companies feel they already spend too much on pain patients; to them, pain treatment is a black hole of expense. They feel there is a good chance the pain patient will move on to a different insurance program in the near future, so there's no need for them to solve long-term problems, no matter how powerful the impact on society. If the lack of proper care means a person can't return to work and must go on disability, that's fine with an insurance company: the cost and responsibility then shifts to the disability system and becomes the taxpayers' problem and expense.

Many insurance companies, health plans, and state workers' compensation departments have hired outside "review physicians" to evaluate what the doctor has done or recommends, specifically looking for reasons to deny treatment. These review physicians, who are not pain specialists, get paid by the companies to meet a "quota of no" by denying claim after claim. Other insurance companies take a different approach, developing multiple layers of administration that doctors must work through to get approval. But the process is so difficult and time-consuming, with the insurance companies putting up so many roadblocks, that most doctors follow the path of least resistance and go back to the pills and injections, or anything else that will be covered.

This might be all right if the covered therapies truly helped. But if they did, would 100 million Americans still be suffering from pain and all of its associated ills? Our health system is supposed to be driven by science, but there are no scientific studies showing, for example, that long-term use of opioids is an effective treatment for chronic pain. I would argue that prescribing pain pills, now a common treatment strategy, took hold through clever marketing and sales work.

Patients have long been kept in the dark as to the effectiveness and the dangers of certain pain relief strategies. For example, studies have shown that the sleeping pills commonly prescribed for insomnia can be seriously dangerous over the long run. Yet how often are patients informed that the use of sleeping pills, even intermittently, is associated with a lower life expectancy? Cognitive-behavioral therapy has been shown to be more effective and much safer than sleeping medications, yet insurance companies rarely cover it. In short, our healthcare system is geared toward quick fixes for pain, so we rely primarily on prescriptions and injections, even though they may not be the best solutions.

Today's pain specialists provide their patients with a lot of interventional or invasive procedures. And that's because insurance pays doctors more when they do some sort of procedure, as opposed to simply educating their patients. A procedure, then, is more profitable than a simple office visit/consultation. Some pain specialists have found they can optimize their cash flow by setting up their own procedure room or surgery center. Then, when they perform a procedure, they get two fees: the professional fee for the procedure, and the facility fee. Meanwhile, many hospitals court doctors who do a lot of procedures, offering them financially advantageous terms if they will move to the hospital and bring their patients with them. While all of this may be legal, the point is financial incentives may not always coincide with the areas where we get the best results.

Here's another fact not known by most patients: Many spinal fusion hardware makers have set up special deals with doctors, allowing them to buy hardware from the company at a discount, then sell it to the hospital where they will be performing the surgery at full price (of course). During the surgery, the doctor will insert the same hardware into the patient that he just made a profit on. Thus, he is paid twice: for performing the surgery and for selling the hardware to the hospital. And, if he happens to have a financial interest in the hospital, he will make even more money.

Whenever extra payments are involved, you have to wonder if the incentive for profit might be clouding the doctor's judgment.

FOLLOW THE MONEY!

Companies that manufacture medications and medical devices have long sought to develop financial relationships with doctors, especially "thought leaders" whom other doctors look to when deciding how to treat patients. To foster these relationships, they offer physicians fees for speaking to other doctors and for conducting research. In these ways, some physicians make tens or even hundreds of thousands of dollars a year, above and beyond what they make practicing medicine.

Up until recently, this flow of money has been impossible to track. But the Affordable Care Act (Obama Care) requires these companies to publicly disclose any and all payments made to doctors of $10 or more. For the first time ever, this information is being collected and put into a national database. It currently shows that during the last five months of 2013, doctors and teaching hospitals in the United States received $3.5 billion from pharmaceutical and medical device companies. This money was spread among nearly 550,000 physicians and more than 1,300 teaching hospitals.

Of course, the fact that a company has paid money to a doctor doesn't necessarily mean that something is amiss. It takes a lot of money to conduct research and keep doctors up to date with the latest knowledge in medicine. So the companies that fund this are doing the nation a service. But when so much money is given to so many doctors, you have to wonder how much and in which ways it is affecting the way that they practice.

The sad truth is that the treatment of pain is often driven by money: If you want to understand why certain things are the way they are, just follow the money. Ask yourself who is profiting and you'll often understand why things are done the way they are. In many cases, the system works well and people suffering from a variety of illnesses and other problems are healed. But the way money flows through the healthcare system doesn't necessarily produce the best pain treatment or support evidence-based treatments like comprehensive, mind–body programs for chronic pain. Instead, the economics support the use of medicines, short-term "solutions," quick follow-ups, sending patients to specialists, and an overdependence on procedures and surgeries that have not been proven effective in the long run. But when a disease becomes a $600 billion industry with lots of special interests profiting off of other peoples' pain, change can be hard to come by. I am sorry to tell you that in our current system there is no financial incentive to get people well.

Doctors are under pressure to make enough money to support their practices and please their patients, who can post poor reviews online and possibly cost them their jobs. They're also pressured by pharmaceutical companies and spinal fusion hardware manufacturers, and by insurance companies who don't want to pay for other kinds of treatment. But now the pendulum is swinging the other way, with doctors under increasing pressure to be more cautious about prescribing painkillers. Concerned about addiction and overdose deaths due to the over-prescription of painkillers, the government is trying to get doctors to more closely regulate the medications they prescribe. Unfortunately, there is no national policy or consensus guiding this action.

This pressure toward tighter regulation of medications has changed the nature of the doctor–patient relationship for the worse, as doctors have been directed to perform urine drug testing and enforce tougher prescription policies. It makes the doctor's role more authoritarian, and less about empathy and compassion. I know that I chose my specialty in order to transform my patients' lives, not police them. Yet the government wants tighter monitoring, without insisting on or even encouraging the creation of comprehensive programs that provide better options for people in pain.

You probably won't learn about better options for relieving chronic pain by talking to your doctor or visiting a pain specialist, for all the reasons I've discussed in this chapter. But the techniques and solutions I lay out in this book really do work. You can conquer your chronic pain and get well.

You Are the Transformation

Changing a culture is hard work and requires teamwork. This means that patients, doctors, and health plans all have to be on the same page. Unfortunately, this will take a long time to occur, and you can't wait when you're in pain. That's why I want to help you get off the sidelines and become actively involved in what needs to happen, now! This book is designed to help you acquire the knowledge and insight you need to take charge of your pain and transform your life.

With each personal victory over chronic pain, your individual success becomes much more than a solo flight. You will touch others, hopefully many, and inspire them to get on a similar journey. And soon we will have a nationwide transformation on our hands!

I wish I could give you a single, one-size-fits-all plan, but the truth is that everyone's pain is different, so everyone's program is unique. Instead of a preset, 1-2-3 type of program, I'll describe the various approaches that have helped my patients, then give you a few examples of each, along with some recommendations for learning more. As you work through the different approaches—calming the brain, reframing harmful thoughts, igniting creativity, movement— you'll find that some of them are instantly comfortable and helpful, while others take some getting used to or may not provide measurable relief right away.

That's perfectly normal. Just keep moving ahead. Keep your eye on the goal of turning your "pain brain" back into a healthy brain, continue working with the comfortable therapies, and experimenting with the others. With time and patience, you may find that all of the therapies are helpful, or you'll discover the mix that's just right for you.

This may seem like a tall order, like everything is being dumped on you when you're hurting, it's hard to focus, and you're depressed, angry or worried about losing your family or your job.

Yes, it is a tall order and it is incredibly unfair that our health system has failed you.

But you *can* do it. I know you can, because I've seen many people, just like you, succeed. They were determined to regain control of their lives—and they did!

Let's start the journey with a look at chronic pain, what it is, and how it turns a healthy brain into a "pain brain."

CHAPTER TWO

The "Pain Brain"

It is in the brain that everything takes place. . . .
It is in the brain that the poppy is red, that the
apple is odorous, that the skylark sings.
—Oscar Wilde

Chronic pain often begins as acute pain, the "regular" pain we all experience when we stub a toe, cut a finger, or suffer some other injury. Acute pain is a symptom of an underlying injury or disease. It's also a warning—the body's way of telling you that something has gone wrong.

For example, if a thorn pricks your finger while you're trimming roses, your body creates a pain signal, an urgent, unpleasant sensation that gets you to pull your hand back and inspect it for damage. As soon as your skin is pricked, nerves in the finger send messages to the brain, informing it that an injury has occurred. The body responds to the danger immediately, generating platelets to plug the breach in the bleeding capillary, sending white blood cells to deal with any bacteria that have entered the body through the break in the skin, and so on. What began as a sharp pain quickly fades to a mild pain, which disappears as the physical injury is resolved. The pain has served its purpose and vanishes.

Acute pain can also be a symptom of disease. Chest pain, for example, can signal the presence of heart disease, while pain in the abdomen may warn that the appendix is inflamed.

Unfortunately, in too many cases, acute pain doesn't cease when it should, but continues long after the original injury has been repaired, becoming chronic pain. Chronic pain can linger for months, years, even decades, and become an all-encompassing state of mind. While acute pain can be seen as a fleeting symptom, it helps to view chronic pain as a disease in and of itself, like diabetes and hypertension. Chronic pain—that burning, shooting, sharp, throbbing, aching, electrical, "ice pick driving straight thought my body" kind of pain—can affect every part of your life. It can take many forms—muscle pain, nerve pain, joint pain—and carry diagnoses like fibromyalgia, rheumatoid arthritis, or sciatica. But its presence always feels cruel and unfair, because it is always there.

Pain Is *Always* Real

Until quite recently, pain was viewed primarily as a symptom of tissue damage or an underlying disease. And when the pain continued after the damage had been resolved, or when no physical reason for it could be identified, those who were hurting were viewed with suspicion by doctors, insurance companies, family members, and friends, for they couldn't understand why. And the longer the pain lasted, the more eyebrows were raised. Sadly, those with chronic pain were often labeled hypochondriacs, malingerers milking the disability system, or just plain kooks.

I remember well in my early days of private practice when I would meet doctors in the hospital and the first thing they asked me was, "How do you know when the pain is real?" This always left me scratching my head while trying to figure out how to say, diplomatically, "Pain is *always* real for the person who is hurting, you numb nut."

Fortunately, such attitudes toward pain began to shift in the latter part of the 20th century, as new technology and research advanced our understanding of what happens in the brain when the body is hurting or injured. These advances made it clear that chronic pain is an experience based on phenomenon created within the brain. What makes chronic pain such a vexing disease is that it influences every-thing that goes on in the brain. This means that the anxiety, depres-sion, fear, forgetfulness, lack of motivation, and other problems that accompany chronic pain are also very real.

The Pain-Changed Brain

Until fairly recently, scientists believed that once we reach adult-hood, our brains don't continue to progress in any meaningful way. This idea began to change at the turn of the 21st century, when we developed high-tech tools that greatly expanded our understand-ing of what goes on in the brain. We now know that the brain is able to reshape itself in response to information and events. In fact, the brain is an always evolving and ever-changing organ—in other words, truly dynamic!

THE EVER-CHANGING BRAIN

When you learn a new language, let's say Italian, new cells are cre-ated in your brain to store what you've learned. As your knowledge of Italian grows, more and more neurons are created to handle this new skill. It's as if an area of your brain is labeled "Italian Language" and given over to everything you learn about the language. But your knowledge of Italian is not really isolated in one little area of your brain. Instead, your "Italian language neurons" form connec-tions with neurons from other parts of your brain, including those dealing with words and speech, as well as culture and history and food and everything else you're learning about Italy while studying the language.

This is an example of neurogenesis, or the birth of new brain cells, which we now know occurs throughout life. As long as you're learning or experiencing new things, ideas, or sensations, your brain will respond by giving birth to new neurons, and linking those neu-rons to existing brain cells.

We have learned that the human brain can keep growing and adapting throughout life, and that everything in the brain is inter-connected. Thus, what happens in one part of the brain likely affects other parts, and all the individual changes to the brain happen in concert and feed off of each other. This means that what seems like a small change in the brain can actually have a major impact on the whole brain, and ultimately the body, as well.

We use the term *neuroplasticity* to describe the ability of the brain to reshape itself, "neuro" referring to the brain, and "plasticity" meaning moldable. You may have witnessed the effects of neuroplas-ticity first-hand. Perhaps your grandfather suffered a stroke and was unable to talk because the areas of his brain handling speech had been heavily damaged. Over time, however, with the aid of a speech thera-pist, your grandfather "re-learned" to speak. As he went through the various exercises provided by the therapist, his brain reshaped itself, with the speech center rerouting its functions around the damaged area. This is neuroplasticity in action. You also enjoy the effects of neuroplasticity every time you learn something new or have a new experience, whether it's algebra, a sport, listening to a new kind of music, or anything else. The brain physically changes itself, even if it's just a tiny bit, to accommodate the new information. However, creating significant neuroplastic changes takes time and repetition, which is why recovering from a stroke can be a long process.

Unfortunately, the process of neuroplasticity doesn't always produce a happy ending. In response to persistent pain, the brain reshapes itself in ways that fuel the pain and create additional prob-lems, such as mood swings and a loss of motivation. We're just begin-ning to understand these changes in the architecture of the chronic "pain brain," but what we've learned so far is an eye-opener. For example, we now know that persistent pain can trigger measureable physical changes in the brain, decreasing the volume of gray matter over the course of a single year of pain.[1] This is a major concern, as a great deal of information is processed in the gray matter, home to the central bodies of neurons and their branched "antennae." Loss of gray matter, which occurs naturally with aging, can hamper thought-processing and decision-making. Studies have shown that persistent pain is associated with advanced reductions in gray matter, which means that chronic pain can literally "age" you.

Neuroscientist Vania Apkarian of Northwestern University has been studying the effects of pain on the brain for many years. He's made many fascinating and disturbing discoveries, including showing significant reductions in the volume of gray matter in patients with chronic low back pain—comparable to an additional ten to 20 years of normal aging. New insights from recently published research conducted in Norway make it clear that:

- About 20 percent of the chronic pain patients studied showed signs of significant impairment in basic cognitive functioning.
- Cognitive problems are more likely to be seen in patients with generalized pain problems or neuropathic pain (pain from nerve dysfunction), as opposed to pain localized to a specific body part.
- Declines in cognitive function in pain patients occurred at the same rate, whether the patients took pain medication or not.

Chronic pain can also trigger alterations to the brain's white matter, which contains the glial cells and myelinated nerve axons that pass signals from one region of the cerebrum to another. Glial cells provide support and nutrition for the neurons, as well as performing "housekeeping" functions such as clearing away debris and excess material. The myelinated nerve axons are covered with myelin, a white, fatty "sheath" that helps speed the transmission of impulses through the nerves. Serious problems such as multiple sclerosis can arise if the myelin sheath is degraded.

If you compare the human brain to a computer, you can think of the gray matter as the central processing unit where decisions are made, while the white matter is the cables, cords, and wires linking everything together. Here's what can happen to your "cables and cords" when chronic pain strikes.

White Matter "Pain Pattern"—For a recent study[2] sponsored by the National Institutes of Health, pain researcher Vania Apkarian, PhD, and his colleagues worked with 46 people who had suffered from low back pain for roughly three months before coming to the hospital for treatment. Dr. Apkarian and his team scanned the patients' brains, using a technique called DTI (diffusion tensor imaging), a form of MRI (magnetic resonance imaging) that allows researchers to study the "architecture" of the brain's white matter, visualizing its structure and integrity down to the microstructural level. The researchers also tracked the volunteers' pain levels over the course of a year.

By the end of the year, about half of the patients had recovered, while the other half continued to suffer from low back pain. The big surprise was that the DTI brain scans showed clear and consistent differences in the white matter between those who recovered and those who continued to suffer pain! Not only that, the white matter of those who continued to suffer looked quite a bit like the white matter of people who were known to suffer from chronic pain.

Here was striking evidence that the brain changes physically when pain settles in—and that an accurate prediction of who would continue to suffer could be made just by looking at the white matter!

Not only is the brain physically altered by chronic pain, there are also changes in the way it functions.

Chronic Pain Alters Brain Blood Flow—In 2008, a scientific study[3] funded by the National Institutes of Health used fMRI (functional magnetic resonance imaging) to track the blood flow through various parts of the brain. Since blood flow increases to parts of the brain that are active, fMRI allows researchers to see which parts are in use at any given moment.

Two groups of volunteers—people suffering from chronic back pain, and healthy people who were not in pain—were asked to perform a simple visual attention task. It wasn't difficult to do, but it required the use of certain areas of the brain. While the volunteers were performing the task, the researchers used the fMRI to measure blood flow to their brains to see which parts were activated and which were "at rest."

You would expect the fMRIs of the chronic pain group and the healthy control group to be similar, because everyone was performing the same task, requiring activation of the same part of the brain. But there were distinct differences in the blood flow through the brains of the pain patients and the healthy comparisons. Specifically, parts of the brain in the chronic pain patients that should have been "at rest" during the task remained active. So even though those in the chronic pain group performed the task as well as the others, their brains behaved differently.

Studies like these paint a picture of how the brains of chronic pain patients are functionally different than those of healthy people. Indeed, the researchers noted that "these findings suggest that the brain of a chronic pain patient is not simply a healthy brain processing pain information, but rather is altered by the persistent pain in a manner reminiscent of other neurological conditions associated with cognitive impairments."

Since the brain controls emotions, sleep, and other behaviors, these may also be affected by chronic pain. Indeed, people in chronic pain are known to suffer from increased depression, anxiety, sleep difficulties, and "fuzzy thinking," as well as a decreased quality of life.[4] They also tend to suffer from a lack of motivation. For example, no matter how often their doctors, therapists, families, and friends encourage them to exercise, many people in chronic pain just can't seem to make themselves do it. Often, just getting through the day is a struggle for them. Until recently, we had no idea why chronic pain patients suffered from a lack of motivation, "fuzzy thinking," and other problems, and we had no way of connecting these problems to the pain. But that's all changing, now that researchers have discovered links between chronic pain and specific parts of the brain, like the following:

Chronic Pain Dampens the Motivation Centers of the Brain—In a fascinating study conducted by Stanford University researchers,[5] laboratory mice were trained to poke their noses through a certain hole in their cages when they were hungry. At the beginning of the study, it only took one nose poke to be rewarded with a food pellet. Over time, the mice had to poke their noses through the hole more and more often to get the food. In other words, it became increasingly difficult and required more motivation to get the food.

After the mice had learned to poke their noses through the hole to get food, the researchers turned some of them into "chronic pain patients" by damaging a paw. Within a week after the pain began, the "chronic pain mice" were less and less likely to work hard for food, compared to the healthy mice. Even when the "chronic pain mice" were given pain medication and could move about easily, they continued to be less motivated and less likely to work for their food.

To find out why, the researchers examined the mice brains and discovered that chronic pain had triggered permanent alterations in the nucleus accumbens, a part of the brain that motivates us do things that improve our chances of survival, and to avoid things that hamper those chances.

Here was solid proof that chronic pain can alter specific regions of the brain and produce harmful results. To make matters worse, in addition to altering the brain physically and functionally, chronic pain can hamper its ability to adapt in helpful ways.

Chronic Pain Slows Learning—Australian researchers asked a group of people suffering from chronic tension-type headaches (CTTH) to perform a learning task in which they moved their thumbs in a specified direction as rapidly as possible.[6] Typically, when people are asked to do this, they get better at it with practice, and the adaptations of the brain as it masters this skill can be tracked. However, the chronic pain patients did not improve their ability to perform the skill, and there were no changes in their brains, suggesting that their brains were unable to adapt sufficiently to master the new skill. This study demonstrates that chronic pain can slow or otherwise interfere with the positive process of neuroplasticity.

We still have a lot to learn, but this much is certain: Chronic pain is not a simple matter of the brain sending out too many "Danger, there's a problem with your back!" messages, like a phone that keeps ringing because some wires have been crossed somewhere in the system. With chronic pain, the brain has truly changed, and significantly so. It has physically reorganized itself around the experience of pain, and is literally compelled to keep that pain alive. It's become a "pain brain."

GENETIC CHANGES PLAY A KEY ROLE

Neuroplastic pain changes to the brain don't happen in isolation. Rather, they are heavily influenced by what is perceived by the body through chemical inflammatory mediators.

Fascinating research has shown that the way genes are expressed can have a big impact on chronic pain, even though there are no changes in the actual DNA sequences. This is known as epigenetics, the study of how certain genes are "turned on" or "turned off," sometimes with negative results. Certain inflammatory mediators can lead to epigenetic changes in the way DNA is expressed or "used" by the body. As a result, environmental factors like stress, nutrition, toxins, medications, and exercise can have a potentially significant impact on a person's pain experience, for better or for worse.

Preliminary studies suggest chronic pain states are associated with widespread epigenetic changes in the brain. For example, in the prefrontal cortex, the amount of change correlates with the severity of the pain. Learning more about the ways in which pain influences epigenetics will help us better understand how the "pain brain" is developed and how it can be healed.

Zeroing In on the Brain Changes

Remember Heather, the 32-year-old woman who developed chronic pain after smashing into a fence while playing softball? My guess is that her brain had been radically altered.

There were undoubtedly changes within Heather's *somatosensory cortex*, the center for receiving sensory information from the body that has a detailed "map" telling the brain where the information is coming from. Imagine cutting a short length of ribbon, placing one end on your left ear and running it over the top of your head to your right ear. This will give you a rough idea of where the somatosensory cortex lies: under the ribbon. The cortex works well until chronic pain sets in, when it becomes altered. Changes in the somatosensory cortex lead to problems in distinguishing where sensory information is coming from, and produce body image distortions that make a painful body part seem larger than it actually is. Changes to the cortex might lead to a dissociation from, or a neglect of, the painful body part, leading the person to ignore a painful body part or avoid using it. This was certainly true in Heather's case. Not only was she so fearful of hitting her injured head that she had nightmares about it, but she didn't want to be touched at all.

Meanwhile the *glial cells*, which are intertwined with and nurture the brain's neurons, can have their own response to ongoing pain. These "helper cells" normally secrete substances that regulate the flow of information from neuron to neuron, increasing or dampening the flow as necessary. But when neurons start firing off lots of pain signals, the glial cells may interpret this as meaning the neurons have been damaged. Attempting to fix the problem, the glial cells secrete substances that allow nerve signals to travel more freely, as well as substances that encourage inflammation, part of the body's healing process. The glial cells are well-intended, but the result of their action is to keep the pain signals flowing and lock the chronic pain patient's brain in a constant state of alarm—which leads to more pain. New research supports the idea that chronic pain may be related to disturbances in the way glial cells and neurons interact,[7] and that disturbed glial cells may keep the pain alive.

It's not just the parts of the brain handling the physical sensations of pain that are altered by chronic pain; so are the areas dealing with the way that pain is understood. As Heather, and everyone else in chronic pain knows, the pain is not just a physical phenomenon. Instead, it is linked to feelings of fear, anxiety, depression, and more. Pain is no longer a solo sensation; it is always accompanied by unhappy feelings: thus Heather's depression, anxiety, and irritability.

There is a special part of the brain where pain is given emotional significance, linking it to fear, depression, and other negative feelings. When Heather first ran into the fence, the feeling of pain passed through this part of her brain, called the *amygdala*, which consists of two almond-shaped areas deep within the organ, one on the right side and one on the left. At first, her pain was linked to feelings of fear and danger: Something bad has happened, get away, get help! Over time, however, as the pain continued, the behavior of Heather's amygdala evolved and it began linking negative emotions to the ongoing pain, leading to personality changes. The pain was initially linked to a feeling of fear, but then it became linked to anger, depression, and other negative feelings. That was why Heather was so angry and grouchy, and snapped at her husband and kids all the time.

The amygdala works closely with an area of the brain called the *prefrontal cortex*, which sits right behind the forehead and handles decision making, social interaction, and planning. Special brain scans have shown that the part of the prefrontal cortex where decision making occurs can shrink in size when chronic pain settles in, explaining why it becomes so difficult to think things through. It's not just that the feeling of pain is so darn distracting: The pain actually makes it harder to think things through and make a decision. Since the prefrontal cortex is our "executive director" and "lead decision maker," changes to this part of the brain may explain changes in Heather's behavior, like avoiding interaction with others and not wanting to do anything but sit.

Close to the amygdala is an area of the brain called the *hippocampus,* which regulates learning and memory. Changes to this area can make it difficult to remember and learn new things. Like the prefrontal cortex, the hippocampus literally shrinks in people suffering from chronic pain,[8] which helps explain why Heather was constantly taking notes at work and forgetting what had just been said. It was impossible for her to remember things the way she had before her injury.

Imagine those pain sensations emanating from Heather's head, neck, and shoulders, triggering feelings of anger and fear, dampening her ability to make decisions and remember, and turning her into "a totally different person." That's all bad enough, but there's more. The continuing pain also changes the way she responds to stress. You may have heard of the "fight or flight response." When something potentially dangerous happens—for example, a speeding car, aimed right at you, appears out of nowhere—specialized areas of your brain respond by pumping out hormones that raise your heart rate, send extra blood to your muscles, and otherwise get you ready to fight—or run—for your life. This is only supposed to happen occasionally, when real danger arises. But chronic pain changes the behavior of the specialized "fight or flight" area of the brain, called the *hypothalamus-pituitary-adrenal axis.* The adrenaline level rises, and as the stress response continues, so does the level of cortisol, the body's major stress hormone. That's why Heather feels like she's "on edge" so often; her body is constantly preparing her to fight or run for her life, even when there's no danger.

These alterations to Heather's brain are frightening enough. But there are others, including changes to some of the higher processing centers like the *anterior cingulate cortex* (ACC). The ACC is involved in a variety of cognitive and emotional functions. It helps us decide which actions to take and how we feel about situations and people. The ACC plays a key role in reward mechanisms, impulse control, decision making, and empathy. Indeed, studies on lesions ("wounds") to the ACC show they create drastic personality changes. We know that the ACC goes through significant neuroplastic changes with chronic pain, and imaging studies indicate that it is a key center of activity for the "pain brain." So it stands to reason that the way pain impacts the ACC can have a major influence on what we eat, how much alcohol we drink, our attitudes at any given moment, and whether or not we say "good morning" to people on the street.

Another higher-processing center of the brain, the *insular cortex*, or *insula*, actively processes pain information. It seems to play an active role in connecting pain sensations with mood changes, and helps regulate body homeostasis, as well as the formation of judgments and opinions. So when you smell the scent of a skunk and decide it's really putrid, your insula has played a key role in forming that decision. The insula also helps with awareness and may be integral to formulating opinions about the intensity of pain. So if something really hurts, the insula will make sure you know about it.

In more ways than we have yet discovered, chronic pain changes the brain, physically and functionally. It takes hold of the brain, creating a "pain matrix" that keeps the pain turned on—always! It activates various circuits that create a symphony of pain: This activation is often referred to as central sensitization, a way of saying that the pain intensity is turned up like the volume on a stereo. The various brain centers involved in this pain matrix continually interact with each other, perpetuating the chronic pain experience. For example, the amygdala can interact with the hippocampus during emotional stress, diminishing the brain's ability to remember. And both the prefrontal cortex and the amygdala regulate emotional responses and behavior, so when they're ensnared in the pain matrix you can suffer from "ping ponging" changes that each seem to make each other worse.

Pain pills, implanted devices, and surgeries have their use, but they do nothing to break up the pain matrix and restore the "pain brain" back to health. The only way to alleviate this kind of pain is to change the brain. The good news is that the power to heal and overcome pain lies within you. Learning how to work with the brain and body in a coordinated way optimizes your ability to make positive neuroplastic changes. Providing the right environment for recovery is a critical component, and engaging in activities and therapies that take advantage of the brain's ability to adapt to and remodel can lead to better pain control—without overdependence on medications or other interventions.

Solving the Pain Equation

Perhaps the best way to understand chronic pain is to think of it as an equation, rather than a single "thing" arising from some injury or anomaly in the body.

Back in the 1960s, Ronald Melzack, a Canadian psychologist and professor of psychology at McGill University, introduced the idea that pain is multidimensional; that is, multiple parts of the brain contribute to pain and are affected by it. He believed that chronic pain is a multidimensional experience, with a sensory component, an affective component, and a cognitive–evaluative component. Each of these components interacts with the others and shapes the final pain response.

In other words, pain is not a single entity, it's more like an equation with multiple factors. There's the sensory factor, which consists of what you are feeling in your nerves, joints, muscles, and other parts of the body. There's the affective factor, all the emotions that come into play with chronic pain, from mild annoyance to deep depression and rage. It's how you feel about what is happening to you. Finally, there's the cognitive–evaluative factor, or how you interpret your pain, as well as any disability, job loss, or other problems associated with your pain.

If we were to write it out, the pain equation would look like this:

$$\text{sensory} + \text{affective} + \text{cognitive-evaluation}$$
$$\div \text{ your unique body and brain}$$
$$= \text{your unique experience of chronic pain}$$

Obviously, this is not an equation I can solve by dashing off a prescription for some pills, or you can solve by taking a few medications. Real relief can only come from modifying each factor in the equation. And that's what you'll learn to do in the coming chapters.

CHAPTER THREE

The Abaci Plan

Nothing is particularly hard if you divide it into small jobs.
—Henry Ford

Sergeant Shane Savage went from war hero to chronic pain patient caught up in a medical system focused with laser-like intensity on dulling pain.

Back in 2010, while Shane and his men were navigating dangerous roads in Afghanistan, their armored truck ran over a roadside bomb and was blown to bits. Shane survived, but he was left with a severe concussion and 24 broken bones. During the next couple years, the 27-year-old man underwent multiple surgeries on his foot and consumed copious amounts of pills for his ongoing pain, PTSD, depression, tremors, and other problems. These included high dosages of some of the strongest pain killers available; enough to dramatically affect his senses and his mood. Whenever Shane mentioned a problem to his doctors, he was given yet another pill. It got to the point where he was taking 12 different medicines a day. Help!

Despite taking all the different medications, Shane continued to suffer pain and his mood became very dark. His world seemed to shrink as he found it more difficult to interact with others and simply get around. Like so many others, Shane lost both himself and his independence to his pain. "Shane kind of turned into a completely different person,"[1] his wife reported; at one point, he sat in his house crying for two days. Then he tried to kill himself—with an overdose of the same pain pills that were meant to help him.

After a brief stay in a psychiatric hospital, Shane returned to his regular regimen of medications, taking up to 300 milligrams of morphine per day. This hefty dose often left him feeling fogged over, detached from life, and lethargic. Although his family loved him as much as ever, he felt all alone. It's very difficult to feel loved when you don't feel well.

It wasn't until one of his daughters told him she couldn't stand the person he had become that Shane resolved to get off the drugs. And he did. He began by hunting through his home and car to find and toss out every last pain pill. He also found his way to a special VA chronic pain program in Tampa that helped him get on a better path—one that now has him living again, despite all that he has been through.

When I present lectures to other physicians, I tell them that Sgt. Savage's story is America's story. While this brave soldier's story is very dramatic because his injuries occurred on the battlefield, many of the patients I see every day struggle with the same, or similar, challenges. I have seen countless people trapped in the same web of pain, dependence on drugs, and hopelessness because they are not getting better. I have seen too many peoples' lives crumble when they find themselves dependent on others, unable to get out and socialize with family and friends, angry and frustrated at doctors and others who don't seem to believe them—and, worst of all, still suffering from pain.

Your own experiences may be similar. And although it would be ideal if we could erase your pain quickly and completely, the truth is we can't create a pain-free world. Bodies age and injuries happen. However, there is an effective approach to easing chronic pain and regaining your rich and fulfilling life. It's a comprehensive, integrated program that focuses on five core elements that are usually diminished or missing in pain patients—and that they desperately want back. It can liberate you, at long last, from the restraints and suffering of chronic pain. Recapturing and preserving these elements is absolutely the most effective way to manage pain over the long term and heal the "pain brain."

The five key elements that must be restored or enhanced are:

- *Mobility*—Your quality of life is inextricably linked to your level of mobility. The more mobile you are, the more you can engage in an active and fulfilling life. Pain can significantly limit your ability to get around or even to remain upright. And losing your mobility can limit your ability to exercise, work, shop, garden, travel, and interact with the world around you, among many other things. That's why regaining mobility is such a critical part of a successful pain management plan. Movement itself is also important to maintaining a healthy heart and brain—so important, in fact, that research has found a direct link between how fast a person can walk and his or her life expectancy. Faster walking is correlated with more years of life.

- *Interaction*—Pain can make you withdraw from others, shun social contact, and avoid intimacy. Withdrawing from others may serve an immediate need (e.g., you need to rest, relax, and recoup), but continued social isolation will only increase your feelings of depression, anxiety, and despair. Based on what we know about the pain equation, revving up these negative feelings can make your experience of pain even worse. Missing time from work due to pain can lead to a loss of structure in your daily life and further increase your isolation. This unfortunate cycle—pain, withdrawal, negative feelings, more pain—will rob you of valuable mechanisms for recovery, for the more alone you feel while in pain, the less likely you are to feel happy and fulfilled. Positive interaction and the emotional support you receive from others can help break this cycle and lessen your pain.

- *Independence*—Pain can rob you of independence on many levels, and the resulting loss of control is very stressful psychologically. Many people find it very disconcerting to rely on others when performing simple daily tasks like preparing meals, bathing, grooming, and grocery shopping. Your economic independence may also suffer if pain prevents you from working. I often see people who have lost their homes or were forced to move because they could no longer afford their mortgages or rent after going on disability. Just the act of going on disability can make you feel that you've lost control; you now depend on the government for financial support. In short, a loss of independence is psychologically distressing and heightens the experience of physical pain.

- *Validation*—If you're like most people with chronic pain, you often feel that nobody really understands what you are experiencing, including your friends, family, coworkers, and even your doctors. And it's no wonder; there are no blood tests, X-rays, MRIs, or other biomarkers that can adequately explain your pain. You might be experiencing excruciating pain, yet you look healthy and have fairly normal test results. Having your pain discounted by others is like a punch in the gut. Nobody wants the validity of their suffering questioned just because technology can't identify it. Yet every day I see folks who struggle with a lack of validation of their pain.

- *Love*—The most basic fundamental need of human beings is love; to love others and be loved in return. But pain can strip love from your life in many different ways, and this loss can be more devastating than the pain itself. Romance, intimacy, family solidarity, and social bonds can slip away when you live with chronic pain, making the pain so much harder to bear. Thus, restoring love to your life is a critical element to overcoming chronic pain.

Addressing these five elements is the key to successful pain management and the basis of this book. In the chapters to come I'll be looking at numerous different approaches, from calming the "pain brain" to modifying your environment, all of which are geared toward increasing your mobility, interaction with others, independence, validation, and the love in your life.

The Good News

The approaches I offer have been carefully selected from the lessons I've learned from my own patients. Through the years, I've watched, listened, and carefully noted what works, even in the face of the biggest challenges. The results I've seen from the approaches described in this book have been gratifying. Most of my patients have become better able to handle work functions and daily activities, and they live with lower levels of disability. Tests have consistently demonstrated positive improvements in their moods, including a reduction in both depression and anxiety. Often there are other benefits, including the ability to be more physically active and walk faster and farther. And most of my patients enjoy less interference from their pain. That is, their pain has been "pushed to the background" and no longer prevents them from embracing life. And once the pain moves to the background, *you* return to the center—the most important change of all—and the process of healing the "pain brain" has begun.

Witnessing the powerful changes this program can make in peoples' lives is how I get my rush. Now I want to help *you* make these same changes, so you can regain *your* life.

The Abaci Plan: Restoration, Recovery, and Relief

The Abaci Plan is built around individual approaches or "pieces," which, taken together, can literally reshape your brain and the way it communicates with your body. By working through the plan, you'll be able to feel better, become more active, enjoy more satisfying relationships, and reach many of your most cherished goals.

Let's take a brief look at my core approaches, each of which will be explained in detail in the chapters to follow.

1. Finding calm in the storm—When chronic pain strikes, your nervous system becomes hypersensitive. It's constantly in the "fight or flight" mode, quick to flood your body with powerful hormones and chemical transmitters that can trigger burnout, anxiety, and other problems. This hypersensitive state, called "central sensitiza-tion," revs up your body's pain system, overwhelms you emotion-ally and physically, and makes it nearly impossible for you to think clearly. It's as if the sensation of pain has been turned way up, like the volume of a radio. Because central sensitization is so overwhelming, the first step in managing chronic pain is calming the nervous system or turning down the "trauma alarm."

You may be surprised to learn that chronic pain and posttrau-matic stress disorder (PTSD) are intimately linked. Although one syndrome does not necessarily cause the other, up to half of all peo-ple suffering from chronic pain also have symptoms of trauma. In some patients, the trauma and pain begin together, as in a soldier who is seriously wounded in battle. In other patients, an injury may "awaken" a trauma from the past—we often see patients with histo-ries of childhood traumas, whether physical, emotional, or sexual. Although the past and present traumas are unrelated, they begin "feeding" off each other. The new pain recreates the reaction of a distant trauma within the nervous system, which increases the over-all sensitivity to pain. In still other patients, the experience of chronic pain itself may become the trauma.

In Chapter 4, you'll learn about the scientific link between trauma and chronic pain. And you'll discover effective ways of addressing trauma and the resulting hyper-arousal of the nervous system through mindfulness, meditation, yoga, breathing exercises, and EMDR (eye movement desensitization and reprocessing).

2. Reframing harmful thoughts—Thoughts are not just ideas or notions; they are also part of a process that continually re-forms the brain. What you think *really* matters, and it can either increase or decrease your pain. Learning how to set aside catastrophic think-ing, anger, fear, and other forms of negative thinking can lessen your experience of pain. And replacing harmful thoughts with positive ones can actually heal your brain and help you regain control of your life.

You'll learn about the connection between thoughts, emotions, and pain, as well as how to reframe your thoughts to avoid the traps that perpetuate your pain. And you'll discover how to think about your pain, fear, and anger in helpful ways, shifting your focus toward gratitude, love, compassion, and kindness.

You'll also learn how to accept pain as a path toward relief. Raging against your pain and what it has done to you is a natural reaction that may even feel good. But when you refuse to accept your pain, you can become drawn into unnecessary treatments that create false hopes and put you at risk of serious complications. The best way to control pain is to accept the changes in your life, let go of negative feelings, grieve for your losses if necessary, and then move ahead. Developing realistic expectations about traditional medical treatments can also bring you closer to acceptance.

The path to relief begins with accepting the challenges before you, embracing yourself and all that is good in your life, and activating the healing power within you.

3. Igniting creativity—The "pain brain" is awash in harmful emotions that drive physical pain. These emotions (fear, anger, frustration, and so on) are often deep-seated and difficult for pain patients to address or even describe. In many cases, they don't even know they exist! Yet these harmful emotions are harbored by almost every pain patient, and act like hidden bacterial infections quietly spewing out poison.

New research shows that art and music can function as medicine, bringing these hidden emotions to the surface, neutralizing many of them, and helping to heal the brain. Using simple techniques, you can use art to unlock your hidden emotions and reshape your brain. It doesn't matter whether or not you have talent in these areas. Even if you think you can't draw or sing, art can be a powerful recovery tool.

4. Using the medicine of movement—Chronic pain restricts a person's ability to move, no matter where the pain may manifest. Yet the body functions and feels better when it's active, which is why movement is a crucial part of the program. Indeed, not moving can become a source of pain. The Spanish Inquisition prevented prisoners from moving as a form of torture.

Because even simple activities like walking and stretching can help heal the "pain brain," in Chapter 7 we'll look at numerous ways to create movement in your life, no matter what your pain level may be. I'll present exercises that can maintain and improve your ability to handle daily activities and even get you up and climbing stairs, if possible. To help you go beyond, we'll examine traditional exercises that strengthen your core and improve your posture, as well as alternative modalities such as yoga, Pilates, tai chi, and chi gong.

5. *Ingesting quality*—Eating right is important, for certain foods can contribute to inflammation. Excess weight exacerbates certain types of pain, and weight gain is a common problem in those who have been injured, further complicating their recovery. In Chapter 8, you'll learn how to use food to reduce your body weight and inflammation levels and give your body the tools it needs to heal. Not only will good nutrition help repair the "pain brain," it can increase your ability to be more physically active, an important part of the healing process.

Because everything you ingest is important, we'll also discuss reducing or even eliminating your opioid medications, for they often cease to be a solution and become a large part of the ongoing problem.

6. *Re-charging*—One of the most common and aggravating side effects of chronic pain is the inability to sleep. Many of my patients tell me they are tired "all the time," that they turned to sleeping pills hoping for relief and soon found themselves dependent on pills that really didn't help. But now they're too frightened to stop taking them!

In Chapter 9 we'll explore the links between sleep and pain, stress, medications, food, and other things that interfere with the good night's rest that pain patients so desperately need. We'll also talk about techniques that can help you sleep longer and better, even as you turn away from potentially dangerous sleeping pills.

7. *Gaining treatment perspective*—The American health system is confusing, costly, riddled with contradictory advice, and designed to rush most patients through exam rooms, procedure rooms, and hospitals, and out the door. The faster you move through the system, the faster the money is earned, but that doesn't necessarily spell success for you. It's critical that you understand what you can expect, realistically, from our healthcare system.

Consider the concept of ROI, or "return on investment." Because many chronic pain treatments are not covered by standard insurance, they must be paid for out-of-pocket. Given the sometimes high cost of alternative treatments, you'll need to decide, in advance, if it's worth the expense. But how do you assess the value of a treatment? How do you put a value on improved quality of life, or balance the extra money spent on one treatment with reduced amounts spent on another? In Chapter 10, we'll look at ways to answer these key questions.

It's also important that you understand how physicians view their patients and present their treatment plans, so you'll know how to use them and their advice to your best advantage. And it's vital to understand how to evaluate health studies and to research treatment possibilities on the Internet.

8. *Mastering time*—Time is a major issue in the life of a pain patient. It can function as a negative factor, with the body atrophying rapidly over time, and the brain becoming more and more of a "pain brain." But time can also be, and should be, a positive factor, with every moment being another opportunity to heal.

In Chapter 11, you'll learn how to use your time to your advantage, turning everyday activities into therapeutic opportunities to re-enter the world, to be with others, and to build you own "pain relief village."

Are You Ready?

It *is* possible to regain your mobility, independence, social and emotional connections, and self-esteem . . . to feel love in abundance . . . to heal your "pain brain" and restore it to health . . . and to prevent chronic pain from taking over your life. All of these can be achieved while simultaneously cutting back on your medications and disentangling yourself from a costly, confusing, and potentially dangerous healthcare system.

Let's begin the journey to relief!

CHAPTER FOUR

Find Calm in the Storm

The self is not something ready-made, but something in continuous formation through choice of action.
—John Dewey

For nearly a year now, Gloria has been on edge around her husband, Jack. No matter how hard she tries and no matter what she does, she can't seem to help him. She feels guilty, as if she is part of the problem or, at the very least, a failure for not being a better spouse.

Meanwhile, Jack is in constant pain. He used to work as a delivery truck driver, until a tire blew out on his big rig while going 60 miles an hour on the freeway. The truck spun out and flipped over. And although Jack walked away from the wreck, he has struggled with incessant headaches and neck pain ever since.

The pain has changed his personality. Jack used to be very social and loved taking the kids to the park to play. Not anymore. He's become very withdrawn, spending most of his time alone, hidden in the bedroom. He sleeps very little at night. "Too much pain," he says, when asked about it. Gloria tries her best to console him and massage him where he hurts, but he just gets angry and snaps at her. He seems to be constantly on the verge of blowing up. And his drinking has escalated.

"I'm worried about how much Jack has been drinking, along with all the pills he takes," Gloria says. "I'm always tense around him. I don't know what to do."

When Jack is questioned by his doctor, he says, "Sometimes, most of the time, I feel like I just can't calm myself down."

Many pain patients feel so overwhelmed by the pain that they can't function well physically—and in some cases, emotionally and cognitively. A major contributing factor to this "meltdown" is a hyper-aroused nervous system, which manifests as feelings of anxiety and stress, sometimes leading to panic attacks. If it were possible to look at the nervous system of almost anyone suffering from chronic pain, you would see that it's all revved up and unable to rest. There's a torrent of chatter flying between the amygdala, the hippocampus, the insular cortex, and other parts of the brain. Mental and emotional alarm bells are ringing louder and more often than they should, and the parts of the brain that normally say "shhh" and calm things down aren't doing the job very well. With all this going on in the nervous system, how could anyone help feeling tense, anxious, and distracted?

In a healthy brain, messages flow from area to area at a measured rate. There's a system of checks and balances, with some brain structures amplifying sensations or emotions, and others quieting them down. The system is flexible, allowing for sudden increases in physical and/or emotional demands and easing back to a calm, normal state when the crisis has passed. In other words, the brain knows how and when to rev itself up and calm itself down.

But when you're caught up in chronic pain, the brain is thrown into panic mode. Overwhelmed, it struggles to calm itself but often it cannot. And we doctors can't do much about your pain problem until we get your system to calm down to some degree. So let's begin with a look at stress, how it affects the body, and how to reduce its deleterious effects.

Chronic Pain Creates Constant Stress

Simply put, stress is "the experience of a challenging event"—not just the event itself, but the *experience* of it, the way your mind and body respond to what is happening.

Stress can take different forms. It can be physical: Let's say you've just been chased by a rabid dog, which left you with a pounding heart, barely able to catch your breath, and sweating bullets. It can be emotional: Imagine you've been forced to interact with a very difficult person. You walk away from the interaction with a pounding headache and an intense desire to scream or punch something. It can also take the form of a mental challenge: You can probably recall a time when you had to take an extremely difficult written test. As you worked your way through the questions, doubting your answers and constantly checking the clock, you probably felt beads of sweat forming on your forehead and the back of your neck may have tightened up.

These three forms of stress—physical, emotional, and mental—may sound like very different things. After all, during the physical stress of being chased by a rabid dog you're racing down the street as fast as your feet will carry you. But the emotional stress of an argument may arise when you're standing completely still. And the mental stress of taking a test creeps in when you're sitting in a chair and the worst that could happen is you squeeze your pencil so hard it snaps in half. Yet to your body, *all* forms of stress represent danger and are treated the same way. No matter which form stress takes, your body instantly prepares you to either fight or run for your life. Whether you're tumbling down a mountain side, being screamed at by an angry client, or desperately trying to think of the right answer, your body responds the same way.

Fight-or-Flight: A "One Size Fits All" Response

The moment your brain senses danger, no matter which form the threat takes, it triggers a cascade of physiological reactions that throw you into the fight-or-flight mode. In a just a split second, you are physiologically equipped to survive, either by fighting back or running away.

Think of a battleship floating peacefully across a fog-shrouded ocean in an old World War II movie. The lookout peers through a break in the fog and suddenly sees an enemy ship coming in fast, guns at the ready. Instantly, he hits the alarm button and a piercing shriek reverberates through the ship, jolting every sailor to action. All unnecessary activity comes to a halt as everyone who has been eating, napping, or swabbing the deck races to their battle stations. The engineers shut down unnecessary machinery and shift all power to the engines and guns. Messages fly back and forth between key parts of the ship, while other areas go silent. Guns are loaded and torpedoes are rammed into the firing tubes in record time, as the ship rapidly picks up speed, ready to engage in battle or blast on out of there. In just a few seconds, the ship has shifted from "cruise mode" to "battle mode."

Something similar happens inside your body when it flips into fight-or-flight mode. It takes a lot of energy to fight or to run, so your heart begins pumping harder and faster, sending a rush of blood through your blood vessels carrying oxygen and glucose, the body's fuel, to your body's cells. Your breathing rate speeds up and small airways in your lungs open wide, so maximal amounts of oxygen get into your blood to keep up with the body's increased demand. This also helps your body expel carbon dioxide generated by all of this sudden, intense activity. Your pupils dilate so you can see better, and your hearing and other senses become sharper. Indeed, your entire nervous system becomes more sensitive, making light look brighter, noises sound louder, and smells seem stronger. Your temperature rises as your body burns through fuel at a rapid rate; increased sweating will release this extra heat through the pores of your skin.

But not all parts of your body are energized, as not all of them are needed at the moment. You want as much blood as possible to go to your brain and the muscles in your arms and legs, so you can think, run, and fight. So the blood vessels to these and other key areas have opened wide, while less critical vessels, like those near the skin's surface, have been temporarily throttled back, leaving your hands and feet feeling cold and clammy. And because it's not absolutely essential that you digest the remnants of your breakfast or perform routine filtering of your body's fluids at the moment, the blood flow to your stomach, kidneys, and certain other areas has also been restricted. For the same reason, activity in your pelvis and bowels has slowed, possibly causing cramping, constipation, and, in males, a lack of erection. Even certain immune system activities get curtailed, as facing immediate danger is more important than tracking down bacteria or dealing with cancer cells. Your survival at *this moment* takes precedence over everything else.

These and other changes happen in the blink of an eye, often before you consciously realize there's danger. That's why you may suddenly jump out of the way of an oncoming car before you've even recognized the danger. Or you feel flushed and hot and your heart pounds when you're dealing with a difficult person, even though you don't feel that you're in danger.

The Need to Recalibrate

The many fight-or-flight changes that can transform you from a relaxed latte sipper into a fighting machine are triggered by at least two different bodily systems: the nervous system and the endocrine system. These two physiologic systems, in turn, trigger the body's immune system.

The nervous system—in particular, the part called the autonomic nervous system—acts like a train engineer, telling your body when to race ahead with the fight-or-flight response, and when to throttle down. It also controls bodily functions crucial to life that you never have to think about, like heartbeat, body temperature, and digestion. The autonomic nervous system is divided into two branches: the sympathetic nervous system (SNS) and the parasympathetic nervous system (PNS). These two branches are opposites in the sense that one revs things up, while the other calms them down.

The SNS swings into action when danger is detected, flipping on the fight-or-flight response and sending electrical messages through-out the body. These messages speed up the heart and lungs, slow the intestines and kidneys, send more blood racing through the muscles and brain, and otherwise prepare the body for action. The SNS is aided by the endocrine system, a "special messenger system" for the autonomic nervous system. The endocrine system consists of hormones, the glands that secrete them, and the target sites that respond to their messages.

A hormone—from the Greek word for "set in motion"—is a chemical substance produced in one part of the body that travels to another part to make something happen. One of these hormones is epinephrine, which is produced and secreted by the adrenal glands. Epinephrine travels through the bloodstream to various targets, such as the heart, which it then instructs to beat harder and faster. Another hormone, called cortisol, increases the level of sugar (glucose) in the bloodstream, ensuring that there's plenty of fuel available during a crisis.

While the SNS readies your body for battle or flight, the PNS does the opposite. Once the danger has passed, the PNS slows your heart and breathing rate, brings your depressed intestinal activity up to normal, and otherwise calms everything down. The calming-down mechanism is just as vital as the revving-up one, for it would be nearly impossible to exist in a permanent state of fight or flight. However, because chronic pain is almost always a very stressful experience, those in pain can become trapped in a nearly perpetual state of fight or flight. Caught in the storm, they cannot calm themselves down.

The Stressed-Out "Pain Brain"

The stress felt by chronic pain patients may be directly related to the physical pain. But emotional stress is almost always present as well, due to frustrations, fears, and the difficulties associated with constant pain. And when a healthy brain is physically altered and becomes a "pain brain," thinking may prove difficult, increasing mental stress.

To get an idea of what's happening inside the brain of a stressed-out pain patient, let's look at the amygdala, twin almond-shaped areas deep within the brain. You can think of the amygdala as the "integrative center for emotions," the part of the brain that tells you when to be sad, fearful, angry, and so on. It's as if information goes to the amygdala, which analyzes it and tells the rest of the brain, "That's bad news, so feel sad," or "This is good; smile!" When the amygdala is hyper-stimulated, as it is in chronic pain, it sees bad news everywhere, part of the reason that people in pain can find themselves awash in negative emotions like anger, fear, and depression.

Normally, other areas of the brain, like the anterior cingulate cortex (ACC), help restrain the amygdala, making sure that your emotions don't run away with you. Think of the amygdala as a guy at a bus stop wailing that the bus is late. "We'll be late, it's never going to come and we're going to lose our jobs," he howls, making everyone else jittery. Now think of the ACC as a woman flipping through the bus schedule on her cell phone and serenely announcing that the bus is just two minutes late, so everything is fine. "Nothing to worry about, it's coming," she says. Unfortunately, the changes that produce the "pain brain" interfere with the ACC's ability to regulate the amygdala, so negative feelings can flow unrestrained.

Further triggering the troubled amygdala is the insular cortex (IC). The IC, another key processor of pain information, eggs on the amygdala even more, increasing and perpetuating feelings of fear. In other words, the IC makes the anxious guy at the bus stop even more panicky and harder to calm down.

Making matters worse, the stress of chronic pain hammers the hippocampus, the portion of the brain that helps regulate learning and memory. Imagine being in a schoolroom trying to study, with a bunch of people right outside the window wailing that the world is coming to an end. You can't close the window, so you have to listen to them all day long. How much studying will you get done with all that racket going on outside? The same thing happens when chronic pain upsets your hippocampus. Disruption of the hippocampus can be very frustrating as it can be difficult to learn new things, or even remember something that happened only minutes earlier.

These physical changes have been studied using new brain imaging techniques that track the parts of the brain that "light up" when subjects engage in various selected tasks. While we have much to learn about the "pain brain," it is clear that physical changes to the brain make it difficult for those in chronic pain to control their emotions, make decisions, focus, reason things through, and much more.

Turn Up the Pain Volume

Simply being in pain is stressful, for your brain interprets it as a threat and activates the body's stress mechanisms. When this situation persists, elevated levels of stress hormones such as cortisol tax your body's resiliency, causing burnout and inhibiting recovery mechanisms. Prolonged cortisol surges triggered by continual stress also inhibit the creation of new nervous system tissue, slow down learning and memory, and help perpetuate existing emotional distress.

It doesn't matter if the stress and pain develop simultaneously or the stress ensues later: Unremitting stress makes it difficult for the nervous system to calm down. That's why the stressed-out "pain brain" is always on edge, hyper-aroused, and feeling everything more intensely, including pain sensations. It's as if the pain volume has been turned up; there's more of it and it hurts more. This phenomenon is called *central sensitization,* and when it strikes, it takes less provocation to trigger more pain. Your body can hurt in response to simple things like being touched or changes in the weather.

Trauma and the Pain Experience

Trauma is a serious and often over-looked problem among chronic pain patients. Whether mild, moderate, or severe enough to qualify as PTSD, signs of trauma are exhibited by up to half of all chronic pain patients—tens of millions of people.

When pain doctors and psychologists talk about trauma, they're referring to a patient's emotional response to an accident, sexual assault, natural disaster, or any other terrible event or period of time. Whether or not she was physically harmed during the traumatic event, the patient develops an intense emotional reaction that may include mood swings, flashbacks, nightmares, social isolation, and other problems.

As I write this, I am treating a patient named Aaron who is suffering from severe pain in his lower back. He's an enthusiastic gym-goer who loves to throw himself into weight lifting and basketball, and rides a bicycle on his non-gym days. We don't know how it happened, for there was no specific fall or injury, but he recently wound up with a herniated L5-S1 disc that is causing him tremendous pain. It's gotten to the point where he can barely sit and cannot sleep through the night. His brain, interpreting this pain as a life-threatening situation, has triggered the fight-or-flight response. And this has sent his blood pressure to sky-high levels over the past week. But he's not suffering from mood swings or other trauma symptoms because he hasn't had an intensely negative emotional reaction to whatever it was that caused his disc to herniate. In short, he's avoided the trauma experience.

However, I have a second patient, Greg, similar to Aaron in age and other respects, who suffered exactly the same L5-S1 herniation when he was mugged by two big, scary-looking thugs in a dark alley. These two patients have the exact same physical problem, but Greg quickly began exhibiting signs of severe emotional distress. Immediately after the mugging, he went into shock and denial. Soon, Greg was experiencing flashbacks of that terrible event, and exhibited sudden flares of anger and other symptoms of trauma. His back pain has persisted for months, triggering the same continual fight-or-flight reaction experienced by Aaron. But Greg also suffered from trauma, which further aroused his nervous system and made his chronic pain experience worse.

Unfortunately, Greg's trauma didn't fade as time passed and his emotional upset persisted until it became full-blown PTSD. This really turned up the dial on his pain. With his brain and body continually awash in stress hormones, Greg's adaptive pathways began to shut down. His SNS and PNS could not work in concert to rev things up then cool things off as necessary. Instead, Greg was in a constant state of agitation, adding another dimension to fight-or-flight known as "freeze." Freeze is a state in which a patient is so overwhelmed that it becomes difficult to handle even basic daily tasks. Once a person becomes frozen by their trauma, healing cannot occur until healthy brain processing has been restored.

Trauma Reactivation

Sometimes the memory of past traumas stored or hidden inside the brain can be "reawakened." A new experience of pain, an injury, or some other stressful event can "wake up" old trauma messengers, even though the trauma may have occurred years earlier and is completely unrelated to the present pain problem. When this "trauma reactivation" occurs, the person in pain does not actually recall the past traumatic event. But he relives the intense emotional response that it created.

Knowledge of a person's life experiences, and piecing together how these experiences may be affecting him today, is an important part of understanding that person's pain. At my center, we perform a comprehensive assessment that includes an in-depth psychological evaluation that looks at past traumas. These traumas come from many sources, including physical, emotional, or sexual abuse, and while it doesn't necessarily cause a back injury or a car accident later in life, it can significantly impact how a person responds to these events by overstimulating the brain's response to pain, and prompting the fight-or-flight and/or freeze responses. Thus, for many pain patients, trauma therapy is a necessary part of the recovery program.

Chronic Pain Itself Is a Source of Trauma

In some cases, the unrelenting nature of the pain experience can become a source of trauma. Frank was a hardworking construction worker with a wife and three small kids. One day, while carrying some heavy lumber on his shoulders, he accidentally stepped into a hole and injured his lower back. His not terribly sympathetic boss told him to just "shake it off" and come back to work after a few days. He got the feeling that his boss was upset with him, as if it were his fault that the accident happened. Unfortunately, Frank's low back pain continued, making it difficult for him to return to work. Frank began treatment, but his pain got worse and his legs started turning numb. His boss had no patience for this and told him not to come back until he was 100 percent well.

After six months of being unable to work, Frank really began to worry. He needed to support his family and knew no other kind of work but carpentry. He kept thinking about how poorly he had been treated by his supervisor, and how guilty he felt about being in too much pain to work or even play ball with his kids. He was more emotional than usual and often broke into tears. Sometimes when he left the house, he suffered panic attacks. Then the nightmares started. Today, Frank exhibits many of the signs of trauma seen in soldiers who have lived through an enemy attack. If his doctors continue to focus solely on Frank's back, overlooking his emotional well-being, Frank will have a great deal of trouble recovering.

Tools for Success

Pain, stress, trauma, and PTSD all cause the "pain brain" to become hyper-aroused, and finding calm within this storm is critical to effective pain management. Mastering techniques that can reduce stress and lessen fear, then, is an integral step to easing the intensity of the pain and finding relief.

Learning how to calm a sensitized "pain brain" is a great place to start. The more techniques you learn, the more empowered you will become. Many of my patients have done very well with a variety of techniques, especially:

- Still meditation
- Active meditation
- Breathing exercises
- Art therapy
- Yoga
- EMDR (eye movement desensitization and reprocessing)

Let's take a brief look at each, focusing on how they help you find calm in the storm. (We'll look at how some of these therapies can also help with other aspects of chronic pain in later chapters.)

Still Meditation

It's normal for the mind to wander from thought to thought, from present to past to future. You may think about your drive to and from work, the TV show playing in the background, what you want for dinner, where you might go on you next vacation, why that guy at the park was such a jerk, and on and on. As your brain flits from thought to thought, it picks up on emotions that are linked to each one, and may begin to dwell on unhappy feelings, giving them more importance and more mental space than they deserve. During the course of the day, as your brain revisits events from the past or imagines what might occur in the future, it can become awash in anger, depression, self-pity, craving, and other negative emotions. Fortunately, your brain also taps into the joy, excitement, anticipation, and other positive emotions that are linked to your thoughts and memories.

Although all of this dreaming, anticipating, and remembering is normal, it can become dangerous for people in chronic pain, for their "trauma brains" are geared to dwell on the negative. The negative emotions linked to unhappy thoughts become amplified, and the positive emotions associated with happy thoughts are downplayed. This can be very harmful to people in pain, for invariably they will think about their pain, the doctors who have failed them, their financial struggles, the jobs they may lose, the friends and family members who don't believe they're really hurting, and other negative things that have happened—or have yet to occur. Such thoughts increase anxiety, depression, and other destructive feelings, contributing to hyper-arousal and setting the stage for amplified pain.

One way to calm the brain and free it from negative thoughts is to practice still meditation. (Active meditation will be discussed later.)

To engage in still meditation, wear loose, comfortable clothing and find a comfortable place to sit, whether on a chair or a mat on the floor. Close your eyes, take a deep breath, and slowly exhale. Then focus solely on the present moment. The idea is to give your mind a rest from its daily patterns of thinking, analyzing, remembering, and planning and to minimize the anxiety, anger, depression, and other feelings that contribute to your pain. To do this, you'll need to focus on something else, something mundane so your mind won't be too busy but engaged enough to block your regular thinking patterns. Most people focus on their breathing.

Try this: Concentrate all of your attention on your breath as you slowly inhale, then hold your breath for a count of one, and slowly exhale, and pausing for a count of one after all the air has exited your lungs, before you take the next breath. It may be helpful to count to four as you inhale, hold for one count, then count to six as you exhale and hold one count. (The exhale should be a little longer than the inhale because it acts as a natural relaxant.) Take nice, slow, easy breaths. You may find that as you relax you can increase the number of counts for both the inhale and the exhale. But don't force it. Just breathe, relax, and focus on your breath. Stray thoughts will certainly come and go. Don't worry about them. Just acknowledge that they are there and return your focus to your breath. That's all there is to it!

It's amazing how much a few minutes of still meditation can relax both mind and body, especially when you make it a daily habit. Studies have shown that it decreases pain, calms the stress response, quells inflammation, improves immune function, boosts positive emotions, and raises overall life satisfaction. Begin with a daily meditation that lasts at least a few minutes, with the goal of noticing when your mind begins to wander and gently bringing it back to the present or a positive intention. As you become more comfortable with the process, try to meditate for longer periods, and perhaps add an extra session at another time during the day to help you "unplug" or get through a rough moment.

The aim is to become more like the impala roaming the African savanna. One moment she is peacefully feeding on the grass, the next she's fleeing for her life from a cheetah, a predator who can chase her down at speeds up to 70 miles per hour, then slash her open with deadly claws. The impala, who risks death at most any moment from cheetahs and lions and other animals, is propelled into the fight-or-flight response over and over again throughout her life. But once the danger is over, she calms down and goes straight back to grazing, keeping an eye out for danger, but not ruminating over what just happened. The impala lives in the moment and easily lets go of the past. To her, whatever happened before is done, and what might happen later isn't yet a matter of concern.

For animals, fear is a survival tool. We use fear that way, too, but then we often hang on to it; we become trapped by our fear and suffer negative physiological and psychological effects. The first step in controlling unnecessary fear is realizing when it's present. Listen to your body. Notice how fast your heart is beating; take your pulse. Tune into your breathing and notice its quality, especially when you feel stressed or in a lot of pain. A normal resting pulse is about 80 beats a minute. Normal breathing should be slow and fairly deep; no short and shallow breaths. Then do 10–15 minutes of still meditation and see how your heart rate and breathing change for the better—proof that you can take charge of unnecessary fear and its negative effects on your mind and body.

You can practice still meditation on your own, or with a group. For assistance in developing your own mediation practice, take a look at *www.headspace.com*, a website with teaching tools plus an app you can download to your smartphone. Many communities now have teachers certified in Mindfulness-Based Stress Reduction, an eight-week program developed by Jon Kabat-Zinn to help you learn still meditation with a focus on managing stress, anxiety, and pain. Kabat-Zinn's book *Full Catastrophe Living* is a classic and a great resource on the subject of meditation.

Active Meditation

Although still meditation can be very helpful, I also urge my patients to add active meditation to their routines. Active meditation means meditating while engaging in some type of physical movement. Done in conjunction with the right kind of activity in the right environment, active meditation can do much to quiet a hyper-aroused, stressed-out nervous system.

A classic example of active meditation is walking. Focusing on the act of walking, just like focusing on your breath, will help you clear away the distractions of daily living, reduce negative thinking, and calm your mind. Many of my patients like to walk outside in their neighborhoods, at a park, or at the beach; anywhere they can feel safe and enjoy the beautiful scenery.

Walking meditation is simple. You begin by standing tall and taking stock of your body. Be aware of the weight of your body pressing through your feet to the ground, and all the tiny movements and adjustments your body must make to stay in an upright position. Then start walking at a slow to normal pace. Don't try to take larger strides than you usually do, or do anything different, just walk and focus on your body. Start with your feet, noticing the way each foot meets the ground, heel first, transferring your weight to the ball of the foot, then lifting off the ground and striding forward. What sensations can you feel in your feet? How do your socks and shoes feel? Are your foot muscles tense? If so, do they need to be, or can you relax them?

Next, shift your awareness to your ankles: Are they relaxed? Move to your lower legs and be aware of how they feel, how the muscles tense and relax with each step, and how your two legs work rhythmically to propel you forward. Slowly bring your awareness up through your body, all the way to the top of your head. Be mindful of how each body part feels, and how all parts contribute to the movement.

Then, tune into your emotions. How are you feeling at this exact moment? Are you happy? Content? Bored? Angry? Depressed? Is your mind full of unnecessary chatter? If so, can you gently push that chatter to the side and focus solely on the way you feel at the moment?

Even without the meditation part, simply getting out of the house and walking outdoors can help improve your psychological and physical states. Consider your outdoor time as therapeutic, especially if you spend most of your time indoors.

Walking, of course, is not the only form of active meditation. Often overwhelmed by the stresses of his job and home life, one of my patients finds it super relaxing just to get into the pool. Simply treading water or moving gently in a pool provides a calm, safe place for him to focus his thoughts and ease anxious feelings.

Breathing Exercises

Your breath is one of the best tools in the world for managing stress and pain; there is no medicine or surgery more effective at "calming the storm" than proper breathing. Slow, rhythmic breathing activates the PNS, soothing body, mind, and soul. The physical rhythms of your diaphragm moving up and down and your lungs expanding and contracting, coupled with the audible whisper of air flowing in and out of your nose, can be the calming "music" that gets you through the storm.

Imagine you're stuck in traffic, frustrated because you're going to be late. This can easily trigger a stress response, plus lots of negative thoughts. But suppose, instead, you turn off the radio, let go of your negative thoughts, and simply listen to your breath as you inhale and exhale at a leisurely pace . . . once, twice, five, even ten times at a stretch. This simple breathing exercise will do much to calm your nervous system.

Now imagine you were to breathe with intention and focus throughout the day, without out having to think about it. Each inhalation would be gathering in of energy, and each exhalation an "ahhhh" of relief you can physically feel in every part of your body.

Remember that you have absolute control over your breathing. With few exceptions—such as when you're exercising hard or suffering from an asthma attack—you can consciously control the quality and length of your breath. This means you can always use your breath to calm life's storms.

Here are some breathing exercises that have worked especially well with my patients.

DIAPHRAGMATIC BREATHING

The goal of this breathing exercise is to relax the belly when you inhale. Lie flat on your back, relax the muscles in your abdomen, and slowly inhale, allowing your belly to expand. Then, allow your belly to fall slowly as you exhale. If you tense your abdomen for a few breathing cycles, then relax it for a few, you'll notice how much easier it is to breathe when it's relaxed and your diaphragm does the "breathing work" for you. Diaphragmatic breathing maximizes the amount of oxygen that goes into your bloodstream, interrupts the fight-or-flight response, and encourages your body's relaxation response.

Try diaphragmatic breathing for five minutes each day, lying on your back completely relaxed, and focusing on your belly as it moves up and down. Listen to the sound of the air passing in and out through your nostrils. Don't worry if your mind wanders; just gently bring your attention back to your breathing.

Whenever you find yourself becoming angry or tense, try placing your hand on your belly so you can feel the in and out motion as you breathe. Concentrate on your breath; your negative emotions will just drift away.

4-7-8 BREATHING

When you're feeling really over-stimulated or your nervous system is hyper-aroused, 4-7-8 breathing is a good exercise to try.

Either sit up or lie down; it doesn't matter as long as your back is straight. Gently place the tip of your tongue against the back of your upper front teeth, at the point where the teeth meet the gums. Relax the rest of your tongue. Then keep your tongue in this position and open your mouth, holding it open as you exhale. Listen to the "whooshing" sound your breath makes as it passes by your tongue and leaves your mouth.

Close your mouth and inhale through your nose, quietly, to the count of 4.

Stop inhaling and hold your breath to the count of 7.

Now breathe out through your mouth as described, with the tip of your tongue against your back teeth, emptying your lungs to the count of 8.

Count silently and be aware of your breath moving in and out of your nose, throat, and lungs. Just a few rounds should be all it takes to achieve a sense of calm. Then, over the course of a month or two, you can gradually build up to a maximum of eight rounds at a sitting.

Sun and Moon Breathing

This time-honored exercise, which uses the sense of touch to help you focus on your breathing, is very helpful in combating stress, anxiety, and other negative emotional states.

Using your left index finger, gently close your right nostril, and exhale through your left nostril. Then inhale through your left nostril.

Release your right nostril and, using your left thumb, gently close your left nostril while exhaling through the right nostril. Then inhale through the right nostril.

Alternate between your right to left nostrils, gently exhaling and inhaling through each one. You can continue this exercise for up to five minutes. Try closing your eyes and focusing on the breath as it leaves and then enters through the open nostril. Feel the air move through your nostril and down into your lungs.

When you've finished your Sun and Moon Breathing, notice how much more relaxed you are than when you began.

These are just a few of the many breathing exercises you can practice on your own. While you'll find that your mind may be quick to wander, focusing on your breath will help to bring it back. And just making the effort to do so will calm a hyper-aroused nervous system and help ease your pain.

Art Therapy

Even if you can't draw a straight line, you can put colors and shapes on paper. And there's something about letting colors and shapes appear as they will that helps you tap into your emotions, which are often buried beneath layers of subconscious mental defenses. Whether these colors and shapes remain vague or take recognizable form doesn't matter. What counts is that the act of drawing, sculpting, or creating other forms of art can become a "mirror" that allows you to see inside yourself and recognize and release hidden emotions that may be contributing to your pain.

The U.S. military recently discovered the power of art therapy for treating PTSD patients and alleviating their symptoms of trauma. Walter Reed National Military Medical Center offers a structured art therapy program for war veterans who have experienced horrific combat events. Creating art helps these veterans unlock and release dark emotions they can't express in words. Once their feelings (anxiety, fear, anger, or depression) are revealed on canvass or in a lump of clay, they become easier for the vets to discuss and process in a meaningful way.

Although you can certainly do art projects on your own, powerful emotional healing can result from working with a trained art therapist, often in a group setting. Being in a group can energize your recovery, help you process emotions, and let you know that you are not alone in your struggle. Also, because others in the group may be further along in their treatment, you will see that it *is* possible to heal. Of course, when working in any group, it is important that you feel safe enough to share your feelings, and not fear that your art is being judged. At my center, patients create their art in a group setting, working with an art therapist who guides them through the process, suggests ideas for their art, and gently encourages them to discuss any issues that arise.

One of my favorite projects is The Mask, which addresses hidden disabilities. Each patient is given a mask that covers the face from chin to hairline, wraps around the sides of the face, and has eye holes. Then he is asked to paint the outside of the mask to represent the way he thinks others see him, while painting the inside as he sees himself. I'm often surprised at the differences between one side of the mask and the other. In one case, the outside of the mask was brightly colored, friendly, and smiling, while the inside looked like there were thirty or forty sharp spikes plunging into the patient's head. This was the first time this stoic and uncomplaining patient revealed his inner pain—even to himself!

The Bridge is another project that brings up deep, often hidden emotions. For this project, the art therapist asks patients to think about what their lives look like now, then draw their current lives on one end of a large piece of paper using any colors, shapes, or images they like. Next, they are asked to think about the future and, on the other end of the paper, draw what they see themselves doing in the future, or what they would like to bring into their lives. The third part of the assignment is to draw some kind of bridge between the images at the two ends of the paper, and put themselves on that bridge.

As with The Mask, the differences between images of the present and the desired future are often huge and filled with meaning. But the bridges may be even more revealing. Some people draw big, strong bridges, with images of themselves striding confidently across. Others draw dilapidated wooden bridges, with so many missing planks that they have to leap over wide gaps to get across. Still others draw bridges made of frayed ropes, with themselves dangling by the feet over shark-infested waters. When these pictures have been completed, the art therapist leads a discussion, asking each patient about that person on her bridge, what that person is thinking, what she needs to cross it successfully, and so on. (Notice that they talk about "that person," rather than "you." Creating this emotional distance makes it easier for many people to speak from the heart.)

Another art therapy project, and one that is very easy to do, is making a mandala, or circle. Since ancient times, the circle has been a symbol of wholeness and harmony, of the rhythms of nature and the life cycle. Since it has no beginning or end, no angles or hard edges, the circle has often been understood as representing the Creator's perfection. Throughout the ages, many cultures and religions, including Native Americans, Hindus, and Buddhists, have used circles to draw spiritual energy, speed healing, and aid meditation.

When used for religious, cultural, or healing purposes, the circle is called a mandala, which is Sanskrit for "circle." Carl Jung, the father of analytic psychology, encouraged his patients to draw mandalas to help them work through their outer defenses and get in touch with their core. Today, many healers use mandala drawing for the same purpose. Again, the point of drawing a mandala is not to create "great art." Instead, it is used to tap into the emotions, especially those that are deeply buried.

At my center, patients create mandalas by drawing a circle, using pen or pencil, and then drawing images inside the circle. They work in a group setting, with the leader presenting a topic or theme to guide their drawing. The drawings inside their circles can be identifiable images, geometric patterns, or just random shapes. The mandala can be black and white, or any number of colors, as each patient desires. People are encouraged to draw what comes to mind instead of planning first; guided by the theme they are given, plus their own inner forces they are asked, simply, to draw, without judgment. If the drawing spills outside of the circle, that's fine. Afterwards, the leader and group discuss various ideas and emotions that emerge from the drawings.

It sounds simple, but art therapy is a very powerful way to bring buried emotions to the surface so they can be addressed. The act of creating is itself a form of meditation, clearing the mind of distracting chatter, and helping quiet the storm. For some, a breakthrough comes from examining what was drawn, then using it as a clue to guide treatment.

Even if you don't want to paint, draw, sculpt, or engage in any other "hands on" form of art, you can gather pictures from magazines that trigger emotional responses or represent ways that you feel. No matter which form it takes, art therapy can help release bottled-up feelings by making an end-run around subconscious barriers erected to hold those terrible feelings at bay.

You can find an art therapist via the American Art Therapy Association at *www.arttherapy.org/*.

Yoga

Yoga is a great tool for managing stress; the combination of postures, breathing, and meditative practice induces parasympathetic relaxation. And scientific studies show that yoga also triggers long-term neuroplastic changes within the brain, in part through epigenetic changes to genes involved in regulating the body's stress response. In other words, yoga alters the stress response for the better on the genetic level, which is great news. These changes are also linked to the aging process, and may be a way of increasing longevity.

I was drawn to yoga several years ago as a pain relief tool, and one of the things that made me fall in love with it was how it helped me manage daily stress. To this day, my wife comments on the positive impact yoga has on my demeanor; she can see it in my face as soon as I walk in the door. Many of the "yoga regulars" I have talked to over the years frequently comment on how their yoga practice has helped them "deal with issues."

You may find it tricky to get started in yoga if you're suffering from chronic pain, as many of the poses and classes may not be a good match for your particular issues. But be aware that there are many kinds of yoga classes. Gentle yoga involves easy stretches and mild poses that most people can handle easily. Restorative yoga utilizes bolsters, blankets, blocks, and other props that allow you to relax in easy, supported postures that bring about maximum relaxation. For those who can handle more activity, there are also more physically challenging forms of yoga. It will help if you think of yoga as therapy, rather than a group exercise session where you feel you must excel or compete with the others. Your goal is to reduce anxiety, lower stress, and to help calm an over-active "pain brain." So steer clear of super-challenging classes and find a teacher who can help you get started on a simple, basic program that works around your limitations and pain.

EMDR

EMDR (eye movement desensitization and reprocessing) is a well-researched and effective treatment for trauma that helps the mind process traumatic memories in a way that leads to peaceful resolution.

This relatively new therapy uses rhythmic eye movements to help reduce the power of emotionally charged memories linked to trauma and PTSD. The therapy consists of bringing to mind a troubling memory or thought as the patient carefully watches the therapist's finger moving back and forth across her face. Forcing the brain to focus on two things at once—reliving the memory and watching the finger—for several 30-second sessions helps the brain process the memory and reduce its "punch."

EMDR was created by psychologist Francine Shapiro in the late 1980s as a treatment for overwhelmed brains unable to cope with the consequences of traumatic experiences. The therapy is performed by mental health practitioners who have been specifically trained in the

technique. You can learn more about EMDR, and find a practitio-
ner in your area, at *www.emdr.com* and *www.emdrhap.org/content/
what-is-emdr/.*

Moving On

Much of what we've talked about in this chapter has to do with setting aside negative thinking and calming the storm within. Now let's
see what we can do with the negative thoughts that still remain; how
we can reframe them in a way that removes their sting, and replace
them with positive thoughts.

CHAPTER FIVE

Reframe Harmful Thoughts

Change your thoughts and you change your world.
—Norman Vincent Peale

England's Queen Victoria was considered one of the luckiest women in the world; not only was she rich and powerful, she was married to a man she adored. But after 21 years of wedded bliss, her husband, Prince Albert, died at the young age of 42. The queen plunged into a deep state of mourning from which she never truly emerged. For the next 40 years, until the day she died, she wore black clothing and insisted that her servants leave Albert's room exactly the way it was at the time of his death. She also ordered them to bring fresh hot water to his room every morning, as they had always done while he was alive, so that he could shave.

Poor Victoria was stuck in her grief, unable to move through it, unable even to consider the possibility of being happy again. This was unfortunate, for it ran counter to a fundamental law of nature:

Life moves in cycles. The heat of summer leads to the crisp winds of fall, followed by the cold and ice of winter, then the gradual thawing and warmth of spring. Nature has always moved through these cycles and always will; this is part of the essential order of the universe.

We also go through cycles, from joy to sorrow, from success to struggle, from health to illness, and back again. Trials and tribulations are part of life, but so is rejuvenation and restoration. We are designed to overcome; it is how we grow and thrive. Many patients have told me they feel stuck in their chronic pain and can't possibly get better. Yet it is unhealthy and unnatural to interfere with life's journey and allow no chance for a new season or a new dawn.

When you get stuck in negative thoughts about your pain, you keep yourself mired in the gloom of winter. What you think really *does* matter, and one of the most important keys to conquering your pain is to reframe your thinking; that is, to turn catastrophic thinking, anger, and other negative thoughts into the positives of gratitude, compassion, and more. In this chapter, you'll learn how to create the positive mindset and attitudes that will help you heal the "pain brain" and regain control of your life.

For every winter, there *can* be a spring. When you suffer a major loss, it's natural to feel sad and depressed, perhaps even angry and helpless as you struggle through the grieving cycle. But eventually you'll process your grief and move on, able to be happy and feel optimistic again. That's very natural. But if you cling to your grief and sadness for too long, you'll never get better or feel better.

No matter what your current problem, with patience and perseverance, you *can* get "unstuck," reclaim your life, and regain the joy of living. I say this with great confidence, as I've seen it happen over and over again.

Replacing Negative with Positive Improves the Pain Equation

Many pain patients get stuck in the gloom of fear, anger, helplessness, and despair, and can't see the light at the end of the tunnel. These negative ways of thinking rev up the amygdala's tendency to attach negative emotions to thoughts, further "fogging" the prefrontal cortex so that it's difficult to think things through clearly. This makes the pain experience even harder to manage. There are several kinds of negative thought processes that can greatly increase your pain. Let's take a look at some of the most common ones.

Catastrophic Thinking

One day, a group of young men were playing an aggressive game of basketball at the gym. Determined to snatch the ball as it rebounded off the basket, two of them, Mark and Hank, leapt into the air, smashed into each other, and crashed to the ground hard, on their backs. Both instantly got up and continued to play, but within a few days each was suffering from terrible lower back pain. Over the months that followed, both went through a rehabilitation program.

Mark did fairly well and eventually went back to playing basketball with the guys. But Hank did not do so well. Despite undergoing treatment that was nearly identical to Mark's, Hank was never able to play a full game of basketball again, always had to restrain himself to protect his back, and suffered from frequent pain flare-ups.

There was no obvious reason for the differences between the two men; they were both in good shape, with very similar injuries and treatments. If you looked at X-rays of their spines, you wouldn't be able to tell which one was in pain and which was not. There was a striking difference, however, in the way each interpreted what was happening to him, from the moment the pain began until today.

If you asked Mark what had caused the problem, he would say, "I smacked into Hank when we went for the rebound, and we both wound up on our butts. Happens all the time." And if you asked him what his doctor had told him, he would reply, "She said the MRI showed I have a few cracks in two discs in my back. But I figured that was probably just some typical wear and tear from playing sports all my life."

Hank's answers, however, were quite different. When asked what happened, he replied, "That jerk Mark deliberately smashed into me! And that's not the first time someone's done that to me!" As for his doctor's explanation of the problem, he said, "She said the MRI showed I had two cracked discs in my back. That sounded really bad and I knew I was in for a lot of hurt. The same thing happened to a friend of mine, and he still uses a cane to get around."

To Mark, the injury was just part of the game, and the doctor's assessment was just a bunch of facts. To Hank, the injury was the result of a deliberate attack, and the doctor's report was a harbinger of disaster. Similar situations, widely different reactions.

Hank was caught up in what we call *catastrophic thinking,* which means interpreting events in a harmful and threatening way that is often exaggerated. Hank told himself that things were bad and would stay bad—if not worse. Over and over again, he ran the worst-case scenarios through his head, wondering if he would ever get better— *doubting* he would ever get better.

When you're in pain, it's easy to fear the worst and imagine all the terrible things that may lie ahead. With catastrophic thinking, everything bad that has happened or might happen becomes magnified. You worry about everything—that your relationships will crumble, you'll lose your job, you'll remain disabled, and more. You feel more and more helpless, as if there's no point in trying to get better.

Many scientific studies have looked at the relationship between catastrophic thinking and chronic pain, and the results are eye-opening. These studies show that those who engage in high levels of catastrophic thinking are more likely to misuse their prescription opioid medications,[1] and that catastrophic thinking is one of the key factors determining the intensity of nerve pain.[2] Catastrophic thinking also increases the *attentional interference* seen with pain,[3] which is the disruption of the brain's ability to concentrate and perform tasks, making it more difficult to function on a daily basis.

Catastrophic thinking takes you out of your real life and traps you in an imaginary world of misery. It worsens the mental storm, sets you on a path toward potentially destructive behavior, and makes it much harder to heal. It also increases the intensity of your pain, making you feel worse.

Fortunately, you can easily put the brakes on catastrophic thinking just by reframing your thoughts. The process is fairly simple:

- *Pay attention to your thoughts*—Tune in to your thoughts, and when you find yourself thinking about the future, listen to what you're telling yourself and try to analyze the scenario you're imagining. Are you thinking about terrible things that are actually happening, or things that might happen? Odds are, you're imagining the worst-possible outcome. This is not realistic and certainly not productive. Fortunately, you don't have to think this way. You *can* control your thoughts.

- *Remind yourself that what you're imagining is not really happening*—Yes, it's possible that the terrible thing you're worrying about might happen, but it probably won't. And in any case, it's not happening right now. What matters most is what's happening now. If it's not happening at this moment, why allow your brain and body to be flooded with stress hormones? Why trigger the fight-or-flight response, given how much damage it causes over the long run? Tell yourself, "It's not happening now. I'll worry about it if and when it becomes a problem."

- *Know that you are resilient*—You've already come through a variety of problems and crises in your life, and you'll do so again. I've seen so many patients, who had thought they could never smile again, take control of their lives and find joy and satisfaction. Remind yourself, "Others with my problem have reclaimed their lives, and so can I."

- *Realize that you are contributing to your own suffering*—Mark Twain once said, "I am an old man and have known a great many troubles, most of which never happened." How many of your troubles have never actually happened, and probably never will? What you tell yourself can make your problems worse—or better. So say to yourself, "With every thought I think, I will help myself heal."

- *Reaffirm your power to stop this destructive mindset*—You're in charge of your thoughts, and that gives you tremendous power. It may take a little practice and a certain amount of time, but you can turn destructive thoughts into neutral or even positive ones. Tell yourself, over and over again, "I can control my thinking."

I once treated a woman who had suffered a neck injury several years earlier and had undergone neck fusion surgery. Her surgeon told her she should always wear a soft neck brace and limit how much she turned her head so she wouldn't reinjure herself. Always concerned and imagining the worst, this woman wore her neck brace constantly and avoided driving, exercising, and doing anything else that required turning her head. Unfortunately, her problems persisted. When she came to my practice I did a careful assessment and told her it was perfectly safe to stop wearing the brace. I also said that she could do much more involving her neck than she had done in years. At first she didn't want to let go of the neck collar and become more physically active. But I got her to try going without it for brief periods, say fifteen minutes a day. Her success was the result of very gradual changes, slowly building up to four hours a day, then six hours. These little behavior modifications led to bigger changes and, ultimately, a huge shift in how she viewed herself and her pain and what was possible.

Today, she no longer wears anything around her neck, engages in a regular exercise program, and is much happier about her increased independence. And her neck, by the way, is fine.

Fear: Getting Out of the Trap

It's natural to be anxious when you are in pain, to be afraid that something you do or don't do will increase it. But there is a difference between normal, healthy fear and unhealthy fear. Healthy fear is nature's way of alerting you to risk; it gets you to think about what you're doing and to take steps to ensure your safety. For example, your fears of running out into the middle of a busy freeway or jumping off the roof of your house are healthy fears that keep you safe.

Unhealthy fear, on the other hand, stops you dead in your tracks for no real reason and keeps you stuck in your pain. You may be afraid to do your exercises, go to work, leave the house, or even leave the room. You may become so controlled by unhealthy fears that you can't get better.

When you're stuck, you feel boxed in and helpless; you're frustrated because you can no longer do many of the things that used to bring you pleasure, like meeting with friends, engaging in sports and hobbies, or just getting through your work day. The feeling that your body "just doesn't work anymore" can open the door to anxiety, loss of self-esteem, and depression—negative thinking that magnifies your pain. It's a vicious circle: Your pain creates fear, and your fear heightens your pain—which makes you even more fearful.

One way to break this cycle is to distinguish between healthy and unhealthy fears. If your leg hurts, it's perfectly normal to fear climbing a mountain. But is it also healthy to fear walking around the block? If you were hit by a car while crossing the street, it's natural to be anxious the next time you cross a street and to look carefully both ways—twice! But it's not healthy to refuse to cross a street ever again because you're fearful. A better idea is to ask a friend to accompany you across the street the first couple of times, watching for danger, and hugging you once you make it.

The first crucial step in dealing with unhealthy fears is to recognize them. Which thoughts or worries stand in your way of having a better life? Sometimes it's hard to know which of your fears may be unhealthy; you might need to ask someone you trust to tell you what she sees. And you should discuss it with your physician and other healers to get their perspectives, as well.

Once you understand which of your fears are problematic, begin to work to overcome them. Try taking baby steps, which will help build your confidence. If getting out of the house is a problem, for example, start with a short walk around the block. Then, when that seems comfortable, add a few blocks. The next step may be a trip to the mall, and so on. Building confidence step by step will help you break through your fears, and slowly but surely you'll begin to realize what you can accomplish. Always remember that there are others who want to help you succeed. Take advantage of their support! Writing your fears in a journal and keeping track of your progress as you face them can also help.

Anger—Adding Fuel to the Fire

When you are experiencing chronic pain, especially when it's coupled with fear, depression, hopelessness, or other negative states of mind, it's completely understandable that you might be angry. Perhaps you're angry at the person who "caused" your pain, or the insurance companies that won't pay for the treatments or medicines prescribed for you, or the doctors who aren't curing you fast enough, or your body, which seems to have failed you, or the people who don't believe you when you tell them you hurt, and more. You may even be angry at life.

You might hold your anger in, bottling it up, or you might vent on others, snapping at them or suddenly exploding. The healthiest approach to handling anger lies somewhere in between these two extremes; that is, expressing your feelings in an appropriate manner without hurting others or yourself. For many people in chronic pain, letting go of anger is a very important process, as anger inflames the pain equation and makes everything worse.

Bruce, one of my patients, worked for many years in a warehouse job that required a lot of heavy lifting. It was hard work, but Bruce liked his job and was close friends with many of his coworkers. Then one day, he strained his back while lifting a box. When Bruce reported the injury to his supervisor, he was told to take some aspirin and keep working. But the pain didn't subside, so Bruce went to see a doctor, who told him to take time off work while he received treatment. Unfortunately, when Bruce finally returned to work, he wasn't able to do everything he'd done in the past. The supervisor let him go a few weeks later.

Bruce had every reason to be upset. He had always been a good employee, yet all he got in return for his efforts was a pink slip when he didn't make a full and rapid recovery from an on-the-job injury. Plus, he was stuck with a back injury. The more Bruce stewed over how he had been wronged, the more intense his back pain felt. It was just like somebody was turning up the dial on his pain.

As you might suspect, the longer Bruce stayed angry, the more his recovery was delayed. In order for him to succeed with his treatments and move on with his career, Bruce had to let go of much of his anger. Overcoming a serious injury is difficult enough without adding the extra, unnecessary stress of ongoing anger.

In order to break his pattern of anger, Bruce needed to identify his anger triggers and change the way he responded to them. For example, stewing over the lack of empathy shown to him by his supervisor just made him feel worse. So when this thought popped into his head, he deliberately thought about his work friends who continued to be supportive, were concerned about his injury, and had always appreciated his work ethic. Determined to keep anger from over-stressing his system, Bruce also utilized some of the tools described in Chapter 4, such as diaphragmatic breathing.

Fortunately, there was a silver lining to this incident. Bruce eventually found a job he liked even better, that also paid better than the old one. It had been time for him to shift gears in his career, face new challenges, and reap new rewards. But Bruce could never have taken advantage of these new opportunities until he processed his anger and allowed himself to move on.

Learned Helplessness and Resiliency

Imagine a little box with a metal plate on the bottom, through which an electric shock can be delivered. You put a mouse in that box and shock him every so often. Because the electric jolt is painful, he tries to get away by running from one side of the box to the other, then back to the center, searching for a safe place. But no matter where he goes, he gets zapped. So soon, he stops trying. He just stands there and takes it. You have just taught him to be helpless.

Several decades ago, Martin Seligman, a psychologist at the University of Pennsylvania, began researching this phenomenon, known as "learned helplessness." His findings, which have been confirmed by many studies, demonstrated that when people believe they have no control over their situation, they tend to give up. Rather than fighting to regain control, or trying a new path, idea, concept, or treatment, they just give up. They have learned to be helpless.

When pain patients developed learned helplessness, they strongly doubt there is any hope for them. "Don't bother trying to get better," they tell themselves. "There's no point." So they stop doing their exercises, give up on their programs, and otherwise surrender to their situations. Just about every week, at least one of my patients tells me he can't engage in some activity, or something won't work, because of his pain. You, too, may feel that way. But just because your shoulder hurt the last five times you tried to play catch with your kids doesn't mean you can't find a way to do it, especially if this activity is really important to you. Perhaps your treatment team can delve deeper into the ball-tossing mechanics, and identify certain muscles that aren't performing quite right at the moment. If a safe and reasonable plan can be developed to help you play catch, you need to be open to that opportunity and give it a chance. This doesn't mean you'll be throwing 90 mile per hour fastballs, but you can still find plenty of satisfaction in throwing the ball around with your kids.

Learned helplessness is the opposite of resiliency, the ability to withstand difficulties, whether physical or emotional. Instead of feeling helpless, the resilient person understands that this is a "season" to get through. He's open to doubling down on what he's been doing, or trying new approaches, in the belief that things will get better, sooner or later. Resilience is problem solving and adapting to achieve positive change and meaningful results. It's a mindset, a willingness to work through problems, instead of just giving up.

Like helplessness, resilience can also be learned. It increases as you meet and overcome challenges, learn to communicate with others effectively, develop good self-management skills, and discover more about yourself and life in general. Resilience can be strengthened by having close family relationships and friendships, being willing to seek help when needed, offering help to others when they are in need, and learning to manage strong feelings and impulses. It increases when you develop healthy tools for dealing with stress, and stay away from alcohol and drug abuse, and other problem behaviors. The ability to find positive meaning in your life in spite of hardships is also important to resilience. And you must firmly believe that you are *not* a helpless victim of circumstance. Those who are resilient refuse to remain stuck in a winter of pain.

Becoming more resilient doesn't mean you'll never be worried, fearful, or otherwise distressed. But it does mean that you'll be able to keep these emotions in check and forge ahead through the difficult times. Embrace these tools for building resiliency:

- *Find meaning in adversity*—Instead of wondering why is life is giving you problems, be thankful you have the opportunity to explore your inner self and become stronger as you learn new ways to connect with yourself, others, and life itself.
- *Build optimism*—Choose to be optimistic. You can do this by paying attention to your thoughts, then focusing on those that are positive and hopeful. Concentrate on the good things that have happened to you, the ways

you've helped others, and the many things you're looking forward to. When you think about the wonderful things to come, imagine yourself actually engaged in them, as if they are happening right now.

- *Accept change*—Life is a continuous arc of change; no one leaves it the way they came in. Embrace these changes, even if they seem unfortunate at the moment, as they are opportunities for exploration and growth.
- *Move toward your goals*—Always keep your eye on the big picture, on the wonderful goals you have for yourself, rather than on today's problems.
- *Connect with positive people*—Feelings are contagious, so connecting with people who are happy, compassionate, optimistic, and positive will lift your mood and improve your health.

Acceptance

Several years ago, Spencer was involved in an unfortunate accident while Christmas shopping in a department store. A mishap with the escalator caused the 45-year-old man to fall backward and land on his tailbone, which triggered severe back pain. Despite many types of treatment, Spencer's back pain did not completely resolve. This really started to bug him several months after the accident, especially because he felt others were to blame for his problem.

Spencer was determined that something had to be done to eliminate his back pain; there was no way he was going to let things continue as they were. During the next seven years, he underwent five back surgeries to fix his problems and wipe out his pain. When the first two failed, he changed doctors, hoping someone else could do a better job. Unfortunately, the more surgeries he underwent, the more problems he developed. Now Spencer takes three potent pain killers and spends most of his time lying flat on his back. He lost his job because he was off work for so long. He is depressed about how things turned out, but still believes he can find a doctor who can put him back together again.

Spencer has not been able to accept the consequences of the accident that injured his back. And his resistance has caused him more pain and suffering than the accident itself because it has led to more anger, agitation, anxiety, and depression. Many patients like Spencer make the mistake of thinking that acceptance of a chronic pain problem is a form of surrender; it's letting the pain win. But this is simply not true!

Think of resistance as a heavy yoke on your shoulders. The heavier the load, the more your muscles have to strain to bear the weight. Resilience, on the other hand, can be compared to leaving that heavy burden behind. Acceptance of change, of the ups and downs of life, actually lightens your load. So if you feel stuck and unable to progress, think about how this battle between resilience and resistance may be affecting you. What have you accepted and what are you resisting? How can you reframe your thoughts and release yourself from unnecessary pain?

Daily Gratitude Helps Keep the Doctor Away

Catastrophic thinking, fear, anger, learned helplessness, and loss of resiliency all inflame the pain equation and make it nearly impossible to find the way back to health and happiness. That's why it's so important to replace these negative thought patterns with positive ones.

The idea that positive thoughts influence both mind and body for the better is not new, although it was only in the latter part of the 20th century that we began studying the link between positive thoughts and health. Although we still have a lot to learn, it seems clear that positive thoughts can add years to your life, reduce depression, strengthen the immune system, improve your ability to cope with stress, and even lower your risk of dying of cardiovascular disease.

One of the more powerful positive thoughts is gratitude; that is, being thankful and realizing that you have been blessed in many ways and continue to receive blessings. Making a habit of being grateful has been shown to reduce anxiety and depression, improve sleep, and increase overall satisfaction with life. It also reduces the tendency to respond with anger when provoked, and increases the likelihood of treating others more kindly.

Some people seem to be naturally grateful, easily finding reasons to count their blessings and share their gratitude with others. But even if you're not one of those folks, you can easily learn to become more grateful. You can start by actually thinking about why you're saying "thank you." We often say these words without thinking, just to be polite. But try taking a minute every time you say "thank you" to remind yourself of why you are thankful.

If, for example, you have just said thank you to a waiter, remind yourself that you have had the pleasure of being served in a restaurant. You were able to select food that you enjoy, and perhaps share a meal with family or friends. If you have just said thank you to a friend who delivered the hammer you asked to borrow, take a moment to think about how great it is to have kind, generous people in your life. If you have just said thank you to the mechanic who fixed your car, think for a moment about the miracle of science that has converted metal, plastic, tires, and oil into a vehicle that allows you to visit more places, spend time with more wonderful people, and see more things than your grandparents (and certainly great-grandparents) ever dreamed possible.

Now take it further and start a daily gratitude journal. Each day, jot down a few things you are grateful for. Things that frequently pop up in my gratitude journal include my wife, my kids, close friends, great coworkers, and the privilege of being able to help others. And these, of course, are just the beginning of my list.

Every so often a patient will let me know how grateful she is for the treatment she is receiving and the kindness of my staff. This is one of the best thank-yous I can receive. I've noticed that patients who verbalize their gratitude often enjoy great success in managing their pain. And they often seek out others who are in need of help, naturally taking on the role of mentor to those fighting similar battles. And, I'm happy to say, positive change is often infectious. Robert Emmons, PhD, of the University of California at Davis, who has conducted a great deal of research on the benefits of gratitude and other positive thoughts, sums it up this way: "Gratitude heals, energizes, and transforms lives."[4] That's why I urge all of my patients to develop an "attitude of gratitude."

The Passion for Compassion

One of the Dalai Lama's best-known quotes from *The Art of Happiness* is, "If you want others to be happy, practice compassion. If you want to be happy, practice compassion."

Compassion is responding to the needs of others and protecting those who are suffering or in need. There are many cultural variations in the definition of the word, but for our purposes, compassion is the expression of love, kindness, and caring to those who need help.

Feeling compassion puts you in the mindset of the giver or caretaker. It can spur you to spread humor among the sad, offer friendship to the lonely, and provide food for the hungry. It can also help you alleviate your pain. You may be thinking, "How on earth can my being compassionate help me with my pain? Shouldn't I be the one receiving compassion from my doctors, family, and friends?"

Well, yes . . . and no!

Certainly, you deserve empathy, kindness, respect, and the prayers of those around you. But, believe it or not, the good thoughts, words, and deeds that emanate from you will, in turn, come right back. That's because compassion helps you gain a better perspective of your own situation. Remember that no matter what your own challenges may be, there is always someone out there who is worse off than you and could benefit from your kindness.

As we discussed earlier, one of the negatives of living with chronic pain is feeling that you are less loved. A great to way to invite more love into your life is to feel and express compassion toward others. I often see patients who are working hard to overcome their own chronic pain challenges reach out to others who are having a rough time. People who do this are special in my eyes, and they seem to attract the affection, support, and respect of others.

Some fascinating research suggests human beings have a built-in "compassionate instinct" that drives us to care about and help others. We have learned that the act of being compassionate causes the release of brain chemicals that make us feel happy and content. Using advanced brain-imaging techniques, researchers have shown that the brain's pleasure centers become more active when people receive money, a good dessert, or some other pleasurable thing. And these same brain centers become equally active when people witness money being given to charity! Other studies have shown that children as young as 2 years old derive as much pleasure from giving treats to others as they do from receiving treats—and they are too young to be driven by the social conventions of politeness and fairness!

Just as importantly, the brain chemicals released through compassion can counteract the effects of other brain chemicals that promote stress. Thus, compassion can serve as an antidote to stress, anger, catastrophic thinking, and other negative thoughts. In addition, many studies have shown that compassion can:

- Increase your resistance to stress
- Improve your marital relations, friendships, and workplace relationships
- Reduce your risk of heart disease
- Lessen your desire to get even with or harm those who have harmed you
- Lengthen your life

One of the key ways compassion works is by increasing your connections to other people, deepening existing connections and helping to forge new ones, as when you reach out to help strangers. Such "social connections" have been shown to reduce inflammation, anxiety, and depression, which, in all three cases, can add years to your life and life to your years.

Compassion also helps you take your mind off yourself—very important for chronic pain patients who often spend a great deal of time focusing on their pain, difficulty getting around, problems at work and at home, and so on. Simply thinking about others can help break the chain of negative thinking.

Finally, being compassionate enhances your ability to give and receive love—one of the five things that pain patients want most, and a goal of any successful pain management plan. When you fill your heart with compassion and gratitude, you can't help but love others and feel their love in return.

A great tool to add to your program is the "Counting Kindness" exercise. Record every act of kindness you perform each day in your Gratitude Journal. Research suggests that this will increase your self-awareness and your general level of happiness in as little as one week.

Bringing It Together

Start writing in your daily Gratitude Journal today. The journal should have three columns on each page: one to list what you are grateful for, a second to record your accomplishments and valuable life experiences, and a third to acknowledge your acts of kindness. Write something in each column every single day. This regular exercise can help you transform the way you see yourself, and reroute your path toward relief.

Overriding negative thought processes like catastrophizing, fear, and anger, and replacing them with gratitude, resilience, compassion, and kindness, will rewire your "pain brain" in a positive manner. This fascinating process will become clear as you make a written record of your thoughts of gratitude, acts of kindness, and the unhealthy fears you wish to overcome. As your negative thoughts are replaced by positive ones, you will find it easier to manage your pain, and that, over time, pain will become less and less a part of your life.

CHAPTER SIX

Ignite Creativity

*Every child is an artist. The problem is how
to remain an artist once he grows up.*
—Pablo Picasso

One day several years ago, when my son was still a baby, my wife and I took him to lunch along with her parents. We propped him in a high chair and ordered a variety of healthy choices off the menu. Once the food came out, we cut up the fruit, bread, and turkey so he could chew them, but my son was having none of it. The more we tried to feed him, the louder he howled. And the more he screamed, the more embarrassed his dear old dad got because I was certain he was disturbing everyone else's lunch.

Sure enough, an elderly lady sitting by herself at the adjacent table leaned over and barked at me, "He is telling you what he wants! Don't you get it?"

Being first-time parents, my wife and I were baffled. Our son wasn't old enough to talk. How did this complete stranger know what he was saying? She pointed to a pile of potato chips and told us that *was what he was asking for. It turned out she was spot on. Once we started feeding our son potato chips—the only unhealthy item on the plate, and the one thing we were trying to avoid—he settled down, happy as a clam, and calm was restored to the restaurant.*

Clearly, I needed help in understanding what my son was experiencing and what he needed to feel better.

The "pain brain" can become a dark place, difficult to understand for those in pain and those treating pain. Part of the challenge in healing it involves unraveling the mysteries hidden deep within a person's suffering. There lie deep-seated emotions that are often very difficult for pain patients to address, describe, or even acknowledge. Frightened by these super-charged feelings, those in pain can build up powerful subconscious walls to protect themselves, blocking their awareness of these emotions, which continue to percolate inside. But the negative feelings act like heavy weights, preventing them from rising above their struggles.

Fortunately, what is difficult to communicate in words can often be expressed through other creative outlets, such as art, music, and dance. These creative outlets can help break through subconscious barriers, heal the "pain brain" by dialing down the perception of pain, boost mood, and otherwise reduce the distressing aspects of the chronic pain experience.

What you learn in this chapter can also become a key step to building your resilience, one of the keys to better pain management. In Chapter 5, we talked about how to improve resilience in several ways: by finding meaning in adversity, building optimism, accepting change, moving toward goals, and connecting with other positive people. Now we can add one more important item to the list: igniting *therapeutic creativity.*

Therapeutic Creativity and the "Pain Brain"

Therapeutic creativity is not just random drawing, dancing, or making music. It is creativity with the purpose of tapping into emotions that cannot be expressed or possibly even accessed. Then, a trained therapist will guide you through the process of healing. The creative projects offered at my center, which include drawing masks, salsa dancing, writing songs, and many other activities, are carefully selected to explore emotions and help heal the brain. Later, many patients find they are able to use what they learned to continue therapeutic creativity on their own.

For years, I have observed the powerful impact that therapeutic creativity can have on the "pain brain." Acting or thinking creatively increases gray matter in parts of the brain, including the periaqueductal gray, or PAG. Sitting right between the more evolutionary-advanced, "thinking" forebrain, and the more primitive brainstem, the PAG plays an important role in modulating responses to internal challenges such as pain. Directly connected to the brainstem, the PAG also influences heart rate, blood pressure, respiration, and other bodily functions related to the stress response and the chronic pain experience.

When all is working well, PAG neurons send chemical messengers that cause other brain cells to fire off signals of their own. These signals reach the spinal cord and dampen the flow of pain messages traveling through the nervous system. At the same time, the PAG receives and coordinates input from the amygdala and other areas where events are assigned emotional impact. More study is needed before we can fully understand the PAG, but it is clear that this part of the brain is crucial to the regulation of pain sensations, responses to stress, and emotions linked to pain and stress.

Creativity also increases gray matter in the right dorsolateral prefrontal cortex, an area of the brain that helps regulate memory, mood, decision-making, behavior, and the creation of social connections. We've long known that the right dorsolateral prefrontal cortex is impaired by pain; now we're learning that its ability to function can be improved by stimulating creativity.

Because creativity is linked to areas of the brain involved in the chronic pain experience—pain perception, stress, emotions, memory, and more—and because so many patients improve when engaged in creative processing, it appears that creativity can physically remodel the "pain brain" and return it to a healthier state.

You *Are* Creative!

When I prescribe creative activities to my patients, many are delighted at the prospect of painting, journaling, knitting, or similar endeavors.

But others are hesitant. "Oh, I can't do that," they say. "I can't paint," or "I can't think of anything to write in a journal." It's important to realize that this is *not* about creating artistic masterpieces. It's about getting well. So don't fall into the trap of judging yourself or the things you create. It's not the artistic merit of your projects that counts—it's what those projects can do to heal your "pain brain."

Try turning the clock back and acting like you're a little kid again. When someone handed you a piece of paper and some crayons, you probably drew or scribbled for hours! And you did so without worrying whether you were producing great art; you were happy just being creative. With a stick in your hand, you became Zorro. With a dishtowel tied around your neck, you leapt off furniture and you imagined you were Superman. With a few dolls, you created entire scenes and invented conversations for different personalities.

You were born with natural curiosity and the desire to explore and express yourself. And that's what creativity is: curiosity combined with exploration and expression. So when you find yourself standing in front of an easel with paint brush in your hand, just paint. If you already know what you'd like to paint, fine. If not, let your hand move across the canvas as it pleases. Don't tell it what to do; let it tell you. If your hand wants to paint on the top part of the canvas, fine. If it wants to dip the brush in a new color, great! Allowing your hand to paint as it pleases shuts down the critical part of your brain that says things like "That's not good enough." This part of your brain is loud and dominant. When it's turned off, other parts of your brain can finally be heard.

The part of your brain where pain is felt may guide your hand to paint some jagged rocks, or perhaps a spike driven into an eyeball. The part of your brain where emotions are felt may guide your hand to paint a frowning face, or some teardrops. The part of your brain dealing with connections to other people may guide your hand to paint a fence with you on one side, all by yourself, and lots of other people on the other side, ignoring you.

It could be that the parts of your brain that finally have a chance to "speak" aren't concerned with specific images right now. Maybe they just want your hand to move across the canvas, first rapidly and then slowly, pushing down hard and then easing up, going in circles in the center and then dabbing dots around the edges.

It doesn't matter what these parts of the brain want your hand to do. The fact that they finally have a chance to "speak" is all that really matters. Maybe they want you to create a recognizable image, an abstract image, or just move your hand and arm with purpose, no matter how obscure that purpose may be to your conscious mind.

It's all creative, and it's all good.

Telling Your Story, Creating Your Future

Human beings have engaged in the arts since the beginning of time, creating everything from cave drawings to sculpture, and engaging in singing and dancing. Each of these art forms provides a way to tell stories about things like love, the harvest, hunting, wars, and more. When we examine the art forms of ancient people, we see and feel their worlds come back to life through their dances, poems, and paintings. Art becomes a window into a person's life, a window that might otherwise remain closed. One of the key benefits of therapeutic creativity is it allows you to open these "windows" to tell your stories, and then create new stories, in a way that spoken words alone cannot.

I have seen it happen so many times. At first, the creative activity helps a person express what he has difficulty saying. Working with colors and shapes, music, movement, or other creative medium helps him tap into buried feelings and memories and, in so doing, makes him more aware of his own story. Then, as he begins to feel better and his "pain brain" heals a bit, he begins to use art to illustrate his desires and create his future in ways words often cannot express. For example, some patients want to repair broken relationships, so they focus on creating images or songs about a loving family, or they engage in dance movements that emphasize connection. And often, they find that their family relations begin to improve.

Therapeutic creativity helps you "find" and express your story, then begin telling a new story, the story of a new you, which you hope will become reality over time. Therapeutic creativity helps you transform your "pain brain" and forge an entry into the kind of world you want to inhabit.

The story many patients tell through their art begins with sadness about their present and their past, then evolves into one with a bright future. The focus of the story rapidly shifts from "Why do I hurt?" to "I *am* going to have a great life!"

Get Creative!

There are many ways to tap into creativity, and *any* creative activity that works for you is just right as long as it is structured to help you access and express your feelings. Just handing someone a bunch of crayons and saying "have fun" doesn't do the trick. But as long as the creative activity helps you capture, express, and recreate your story, any form of art or movement will do. The creative therapies I have found most helpful involve dance, music, art, and crocheting/knitting/quilting. So let's take a quick look at those.

Dance Therapy

One of the exercise trainers I work with, Lucrecia Martinez, has a background in salsa dancing, so she began offering a Latin dance class to our patients. It didn't matter if they could move like a Dancing With the Stars *pro or were pretty much confined to a chair. The only requirement was that they move to the music.*

A lot of the patients were inhibited at first, moving very tentatively to the beat—and sometimes not to the beat—but gradually, they got into the spirit of things. They stopped judging and comparing themselves to others and just let their bodies move to the music. Even those who couldn't stand up, let their arms and shoulders respond to the rhythm as they sat in their chairs. After a few weeks, I was amazed at the results, for I knew how broken these patients had been.

For example, there was Eric Morton, who had been accidently electrocuted a few years earlier and lost the use of his right arm. He held his arm against his side, unable to use it. For many years, Eric had struggled with the trauma of his injury, chronic pain, and depression. He took huge doses of one medicine after another, but never found relief. After being invited to Lucrecia's dance class several times, Eric finally agreed to try it. He went once, then again, and soon became a regular.

"The class was fun," Eric said. "It felt good not to be focused on my pain and not to care about looking silly. I had a good time, it gave me a good workout, and I kept wanting to go back."

"It took some time to get used to the fact that I could only use my left arm, so I couldn't move the way the others could. But I got into the rhythm and learned to adapt. It got to be even more fun when I realized I could move in ways I never thought about. I never in my wildest dreams thought I would be doing something like this."

Dancing, moving, and laughing with the others at their goofs really lifted Eric's spirits. A few months ago, when Lucrecia reluctantly told everyone she could no longer teach the Monday class, she and the class asked Eric to take over. He agreed, and now, a man who has lost the use of his right arm and long struggled with pain and depression, teaches a high-energy dance class!

"I go because I want to work more on myself," Eric said, "to keep pushing against my limits. Plus, there are people who want to go to my class. They say I inspire them. I guess they feel that if someone with only one workable arm can do it, they can, too."

"Plenty of people come by and say, 'I see you do it, and it looks like fun.' It is fun. Even if it's just for an hour, I'm not thinking about the pain and the fact that I can't use my arm. I'm using the rest of my body in ways I never thought possible. And above all else, I'm enjoying it. It was difficult at first, but as you keep pushing yourself and reaching new heights, it's great. You learn that you don't have to allow pain or inability to stop you."

Human beings have probably always used dance to tell stories. In ancient days, warriors draped themselves in animal skins and danced around the fire to tell the story of a successful hunt. Later, the intricate hand movements of the Polynesian hula dance evoked both nature and emotions. Fred Astaire and Ginger Rogers told stories of love and yearning through their dancing, while many of today's modern pop stars use dance to describe sexual desire and the urge to smash social norms.

Dancing is definitely a form of therapeutic creativity, as it forces the brain to solve problems on different levels. In any structured dance class, the brain has to perform several functions: watch the instructor, pick up the steps, and figure out how to work around the body's physical limitations. The music further stimulates activity in the brain, which, in turn, prompts the body to move and do things that might otherwise be inhibited by the desire to avoid pain. This letting loose of the body has many benefits, not the least of which is an improvement in mood and increased feelings of joyfulness.

Dance and dance-like movements also help in other ways, releasing fluids that reduce joint pain, improving circulation, burning off stress hormones, and otherwise tuning up the body. Many studies have shown that movement and exercise help reduce blood pressure, boost metabolism, reduce anxiety, combat depression, improve sleep, and increase self-esteem.

And, of course, dance is performed to music, which has its own therapeutic benefits, as described in the next section. So dancing to music is really a combination of two forms of therapy.

Music Therapy

For me, one of the perks of having dance classes at my center is the music travels down the hall and into my office. As soon as I hear that beat percolating, I start to smile and my mood brightens. The tone and energy of the whole center changes when someone pushes the "on" button on the CD player. But this doesn't surprise me: as an anesthesiologist, I often used music in the operating and procedure rooms. And at the surgery center, I try to make sure that calming music is available to patients when they have procedures done. They often tell me that they appreciate having music available to calm their nerves and help them feel more comfortable. In my personal life, when I am working on a book and really need to get with the flow, playing a little Mozart always seems to do the trick.

Music is a universal art form, found in every culture at every time in history: from primitive tribes rhythmically beating the ground with sticks around a campfire, to mothers singing lullabies to their babies; from courting couples snuggling to love songs to teenagers plugged into electronic devices; from barely noticeable piped-in elevator music to joyful waltzes at a wedding.

Given the way music has always been such an integral part of human life, it's no surprise that it has powerful effects on the brain. We're still in the early stages of music–brain studies, but we know that music plugs into brain pathways in many ways, including the activation of the amygdala, hippocampus, and other brain areas associated with emotions and emotional behaviors. Music also seems to play a role in the release of endorphins, dopamine, and other "feel-good" brain chemicals.[1]

More specifically, music calms down neural activity in the brain, decreases anxiety, induces relaxation, and reduces stress. A study with cancer patients showed that music therapy helped strengthen their sense of control, while reducing their pain. We can easily measure the effects of music therapy on the heart rate and respiration, both of which slow down, just as we can see a drop in levels of cortisol, one of the most powerful stress hormones.

As with drawing or painting, the music you create or listen to is not to be judged. Just enjoy the moment.

Art Therapy

Chapter 4 showed how art helped people find calm in the storm of chronic pain. But art therapy can also stimulate creativity in a broader sense—a creative bent you might not even realize you possess.

One of my patients, Brandon, an enthusiastic motorcycle racer, crashed "a few too many times" as he put it, and had undergone several surgeries to repair the damage. "My entire left side is titanium," he joked. But he wasn't bothered by chronic pain until he suffered an on-the-job injury. An electrician, Brandon was standing on a ladder installing overhead piping when he suddenly felt a tremendous pain in his left shoulder. Recoiling, he lost his balance, and fell off the ladder, hitting his back on a metal desk, then flipping over and landing face-first on the concrete. Brandon ended up with a dislocated left shoulder that caused him terrible pain.

"I went to physical therapy," he told me, "and was slowly but surely getting better." But then a physical therapy manipulation of his left arm sent waves of unimaginable pain ricocheting through his arm and body.

"It felt way worse than the initial injury," he said. "I was on a vinyl-covered table and I grabbed that vinyl so hard, I ripped it off the cushion!"

After that, Brandon was in constant pain. He soon ran through all the physical therapy sessions allowed by his HMO, and was referred to my center. When he arrived, Brandon's pain was so intense he was unable to hold a glass with his left hand or open a door with his left arm. And he had to lie down every so often to relieve the pain caused by his shoulder supporting the weight of his arm.

When our art therapist, Christine Hirabayashi, first discussed art therapy with Brandon, he was unimpressed. He couldn't see how expressing himself in such a way could do anything to relieve his pain. So Brandon didn't participate in any therapeutic art activities, except for the expression mask exercise.

"That piqued my interest a little bit. I knew I had a lot of stuff to work on and I wanted to go down the rabbit hole and see where it would take me."

It didn't take long before Brandon threw himself wholeheartedly in the art program.

"It really helped me get in touch with my feelings," he said later. "And the nonjudgmental environment helped me curb my self-critic, the thing that screams in your ear when you do something you think you don't have an aptitude for, but you want to try anyway."

After graduating from the program, he came to a special Friday night class that was open to all, where people can paint, sculpt, draw, or try other forms of art. Lots of materials are available, and everyone is encouraged to do whatever seems appealing. Brandon didn't know what to do, but he knew he wanted to create. Still feeling that a paint brush or pencil was beyond his skill level, he happened to notice a motorized drill sitting on a shelf. It had nothing to do with art; the studio was in the process of being remodeled and the workers had left a drill behind. But it gave him an idea.

Brandon asked Christine for a canvas, then rigged it up so the canvas was suspended from the drill, and when he turned the drill on, the canvas spun round and round. Once he got the canvas spinning, Brandon began pouring acrylic paints on its surface.

"It was a mess!" he said. "But it was a tipping point for me. I liked choosing the colors and pouring them on, depending on how I was feeling at the moment. Right then, I went from being curious about art to wanting to pursue it."

Brandon progressed from his color-spun art to a more formalized version, and today he uses a rake to create large-scale beach art.

"It's my moving meditation around my condition," he explains. Dragging a rake behind him, he walks in circles or other patterns, nothing pre-determined—just going whichever direction his body wants to take at the moment.

"Once I start moving like this, I get into a different head space. The movement becomes more like a meditation. It's a total cathartic experience. When I'm in the process of creating, I'm not cognizant of what's happening around me. But afterwards, I feel like I've moved negative things out of my body. I'll go out here, drag a rake behind me, and let things happen. The art tells me what it wants."

This, however, doesn't mean that Brandon's pain is completely gone.

"A lot of times I have to stop and lie on the beach, or leave because of the pain. I try to be honest with myself, my body, my emotions, and my state of being. But as long as I'm present with all of those, I can learn something every time I do this."

The art has allowed Brandon to help others as well. He liked it when others in the art therapy program began to use his spinning machine to create their own art. Now, when he's creating on the beach, he says, "People see me create something, and it has an impact on them. They come talk to me and tell me how my art affects them. It pulls them out of their automated state, makes them think about themselves. Maybe I'm thinking of things in my life that are not so nice, but I'm pulling in people who are impacted in a positive way!"

Crocheting/Knitting/Quilting

Crocheting, knitting, and quilting are considered therapeutic activities because they require the brain to focus on complex problems, often in succession. When the conscious mind focuses entirely on one thing, pain and other problems fade into the background, which happens to be the theory behind meditation. Thus, the repetitive hand motions used in crocheting, knitting, and quilting can have the same effects on the mind and body as meditation, including a reduction in heart and respiratory rate, reduced stress, and increased relaxation. Yet at the same time, the brain gets a workout by focusing for long periods of time on an enjoyable activity, and keeping track of lots of little details.

When performed in a group, crocheting, knitting, and quilting can also help pain patients connect with each other, and even help those outside the group. Some of our patients have gotten involved in knitting blankets for cancer patients. For several years, our patients have put on an annual arts and crafts fair during the holidays. This festive event not only brings people together, but offers an opportunity for patients to create something that can be used by other people.

These activities not only give pain patients a way to shift the focus away from their pain and do something for others, it also allows them to create a new story about themselves. Instead of victims, they become heroes, creating works of art, blankets, socks, and other items that bring comfort to poor people, hospitalized patients, and our men and women in the service. The stories the patients tell about themselves change from "I was struck by this terrible pain . . ." to "I helped people overcome their problems by. . . ." This, of course, is a wonderful medicine.

From Creativity Comes Meaning

Being creative can help you find meaning in adversity, as your art or creative activity begins to take on a life of its own. It can give you a reason to set and move toward new goals, work with other positive people, and become more optimistic as you witness your own progression. Not only will you make progress in your creative activities, you'll find that your negative feelings will surface and lose much of their power. And you'll find that you are completely capable of setting and accomplishing your goals. You may be surprised at how powerful you become!

CHAPTER SEVEN

Use the Medicine of Movement

It's not whether you get knocked down,
it's whether you get back up.
—Vince Lombardi

Yu immigrated to the United States with his family in the hope of offering his children a bright future and a top-notch education. A skilled chef, he quickly found work in a busy kitchen at a popular restaurant. One day, while he was chopping up some whole chickens, the cleaver slipped from his grip and sliced through the thumb, index, and middle finger of his left hand. Emergency surgery was performed to repair the nerve and tendon damage in his fingers.

Despite a successful surgery, Yu continued to suffer from pain in his left hand and fingers, which seemed to grow progressively worse over the next several weeks. Once the wounds had healed, his surgeon encouraged him to start therapy, but Yu found it very difficult to tolerate any movement or activity in his injured hand due to pain.

Instead of improving over time, his hand just seemed to get more swollen and sensitive to the touch, and it felt like it was on fire. The pain spread up his arm to his neck and became so intense that Yu stopped using his left hand altogether. When he saw his doctor for a follow-up visit three months after the injury, he was cradling his entire left arm to protect it from the world around him.

When Yu looked at himself in the mirror, he saw an arm that looked distorted and much larger than the other. When doing things around the house, he ignored his left hand and did whatever he could with his right hand, which made things more tolerable. He began to wonder how he was ever going to support his family again. The many hardships he had endured to secure his family's future seemed for naught—all because of one simple kitchen accident.

Every day, people caught in unfortunate predicaments like Yu's come to doctors like me for help. A vital part of the treatment for anything that causes chronic pain is recovering the functional use of what has been lost. In a case like Yu's, this can be a challenging and lengthy process.

The "Pain Body"

We have spent a lot of time focusing on healing the "pain brain." But what about the role of the "pain body" in the pain experience? When one part of the body hurts to be touched or moved, the rest of the body rallies to protect and guard what it perceives to be injured. This leads to changes in body mechanics, like cradling a painful hand with the good hand or shifting weight from a painful leg to the other one. The whole body rapidly adapts when pain persists, even if the pain resides in one small area. The sum total of all of the intricate adjustments that take place in response to pain is referred to as the "pain body"—the opposite of a healthy, high-functioning version of ourselves.

Remember the pain equation I introduced in Chapter 2? You can think of the "pain body" as the "sensory" part of that equation:

$$sensory + affective + cognitive\text{-}evaluation$$
$$\div\ your\ unique\ body\ and\ brain$$
$$=\ your\ unique\ experience\ of\ chronic\ pain$$

The "pain body" has the power to hold the "pain brain" hostage, keeping a person in a constant state of pain. When the "pain body" feels broken and unable to free itself, it overwhelms the "pain brain" with toxic information in the form of inflammatory messengers, nerve signals, and immune responses that perpetuate and amplify the pain. Then it's no longer just a matter of the "pain brain" causing pain, emotional distress, and mental confusion: the body adds distressing signals of its own, which makes everything much worse. Fortunately, while the "pain body" is a powerful part of the pain equation, the "active body" is equally powerful, in a positive way. The "active body" has the power to release the "pain brain" and heal the body, mind, and soul.

Recently, a 30-year-old woman came to see me for the first time. She had begun having back problems a few years earlier and decided to have a fusion surgery to eliminate her pain. Unfortunately, things only got worse, and by the time she shuffled slowly into my office, she was living with her parents because she couldn't function without assistance. And she was spending almost all day, every day, lying flat on her back. Toward the end of our visit, she asked me if her pain would ever go away, or at least recede.

"That all depends on how active you become," I replied. "I have never seen anyone who is inactive for most of the day get rid of their constant pain. But those who start exercising regularly and become very active seem to do the best—and hurt the least."

There is absolutely no doubt in my mind that inactivity is an underappreciated contributor to continuous pain; I see the correlation between the two every day. One of the first things I ask a new patient is to describe his typical day, for his answers will help me understand how his body is functioning and how pain limits his daily activities. Here are some responses I hear over and over:

- "It takes me about two hours to get out of bed and get going."
- "My daughter helps me put on my shoes and socks."
- "I can putter around the house, but I have to take lots of breaks."
- "I can no longer drive."
- "I can't get comfortable, so I alternate between standing and lying flat all day long."

- "I don't sleep well at night, so I sleep on and off through the day."
- "I spend most of my day in my recliner."
- "If I try to do a few things around the house, like sweep the floor or do the laundry, then I'm down and out for the next three days in bed."
- "I haven't worked in years. Nobody wants to hire someone like me."

When I hear answers like these, I know it's going to take a lot of work to turn things around because these folks are lacking two of the most important elements of pain management: mobility and independence. And odds are, their physical limitations are also contributing to significant social isolation, which just makes everything worse.

Make the Move Toward Relief

The human body thrives on movement. It was designed to move, not to sit at a desk for long hours or lie on the couch all day. On a physiologic level, movement triggers the production of important hormones and proteins, squeezes blood through the capillaries, "cleanses" and moisturizes the joints, maintains muscle strength, aids digestion, helps control blood pressure and blood sugar, strengthens the bones, enhances the immune system, slows the process of aging, and more.

Having a physically active body leads, among other things, to improved fitness, a reduced risk of cardiovascular disease and many other illnesses, enhanced sleep, less constipation, and better sex. Surprisingly, activity can also reduce your pain levels! More and more scientific studies have demonstrated that physical activity helps improve many of the most common painful conditions. For example:

- Walking, strength training, Pilates, and yoga can all help counter chronic low back pain.[1,2,3]
- Many types of low-to-moderate-intensity exercise, from aerobic exercise to Qi Gong, decrease the pain of fibromyalgia, while improving mood and sleep.[4]

- Certain types of yoga combat the pain, fatigue, and depression commonly experienced with fibromyalgia.[5]
- Exercise reduces arthritis pain, while improving function, mood, and quality of life measures.[6]
- Yoga can reduce joint pain and tenderness, while improving mental health, in people with both rheumatoid arthritis and osteoarthritis.[7]
- Walking helps protect against developing functional limitations in people with or at risk of osteoarthritis of the knee.[8]

All it takes to enjoy these benefits is engaging in regular movement. Who wouldn't sign up for that?

Exercise and the Brain

What makes movement such a powerful weapon against pain? A growing body of research has found that movement helps remodel key parts of the "pain brain." In other words, when you move, your mind and body work together to boost each other's healing power. For example, in just your brain alone, activating your body leads to improved function of the anterior cingulate cortex, insular cortex, reward pathways, stress regulation pathways, and motor and somatosensory cortex. In short, movement helps convert the "pain brain" back to a healthy brain.

There are too many studies regarding this phenomena to describe them all, so I'll just touch upon some of the more exciting ones. In one, researchers from Harvard Medical School[9] looked at effects of exercise on gray matter in the hippocampus in human volunteers. The volume of gray matter in the brain normally declines with age, and this "shrinkage" is also seen in chronic pain patients, the reason that chronic pain can, in a sense, cause premature aging.

In this study, the exercise habits of 61 adults, ranging in age from 18 to 45, were examined, and the volume of gray matter in the right hippocampus was measured via structural magnetic resonance imaging. The results were clear: The more time spent exercising per week, the larger the volume of gray matter. The researchers concluded that exercise seems to protect the hippocampus, a result that correlates with what other studies have discovered about children and seniors.

How does exercise protect the hippocampus? One way is by improving the flow of blood and oxygen to the brain. But perhaps even more significant is the increased production of neurotrophic substances, which stimulate the growth of brain tissue and the development of receptors where these substances "plug in" to do their work. In other words, when you exercise, you "issue orders" to your hippocampus to grow, and give it the tools to do so. This is very important, for many studies have shown that by increasing the size of the hippocampus, exercise improves memory.

You don't have to run five or ten miles every day to get brain-boosting benefits from exercise. A study[10] with healthy but non-exercising adults, ages 55 through 80, found that simply walking three times a week for 40-minute sessions can cause the hippocampus to grow 2 percent in a year. This 2 percent increase is an incredible figure, considering that the hippocampus typically *shrinks* by 1–2 percent every year after a certain age.

Exercise also "lights up" the insular cortex, which is intimately involved in processing pain information. Back in 1997, researchers demonstrated for the first time that physical activity (in this case, cycling) activates this key brain region.[11] We've since learned that more intense exercise has a stronger effect on the insular cortex than less-intense exercise.

The prefrontal cortex—which is involved in decision-making, planning, and social interaction—is also positively influenced by exercise. For a study involving a group of older adults, the volunteers were asked to perform a working memory task both before and after riding a stationary bicycle.[12] Their ability to perform the memory task improved after exercise, and the "before" and "after" brain scans showed that the exercise enhanced activity in the prefrontal cortex.

Exercise even triggers the reward center in the brain,[13] the same part stimulated by certain illegal drugs. But exercise-induced rewards increase feelings of well-being without the dangerous side effects. And the feelings aren't just momentary, for exercise causes positive neuroplastic changes in the reward areas of the brain.

An Active Body Leads to a Happier You!

Not only can exercise improve the "sensory" part of the pain equation, but it can also help diminish the "affective" (emotional) elements. For example, new research has shown that exercise makes us more resilient. In a very clever experiment,[14] researchers from the National Institutes of Mental Health combined aggressive, alpha male mice with meeker counterparts to test the effects of exercise. The alpha males were each assigned to their own cages. Meanwhile, the weaker, meeker mice were divided into two groups. One group was allowed to run on exercise wheels and explore tubes placed in their cages, while the other group was not.

Then each of the meek mice was placed in a cage with an alpha mouse, separated only by a glass barrier. As expected, the alpha mice began acting like bullies and doing their best to intimidate the meeker ones. And when the partitions were removed for five-minute periods, the alphas physically went after the meek ones, and had to be restrained.

All of the meek mice displayed submissive behavior when confronted by the alpha mice, which is normal. But the meek mice who had *not* been allowed to exercise also became emotional wrecks, displaying "anxiety-like behavior" even when the alphas were not present and often hiding in the corners of their cages. The exercising meek mice, on the other hand, behaved normally once the alpha mice were gone, going about their business as if nothing had happened.

To determine how exercise made one group of meek mice more resilient and able to deal with stress, the researchers examined their brains. They found that in the exercising mice, nerve cells in the amygdala and medial prefrontal cortex had been firing often and rapidly in the previous few weeks. But these same brain cells had been much quieter in the non-exercising mice. Exercise, in effect, "turned up the volume" in these important parts of the brain, making the mice better able to handle stress.

It doesn't take much exercise to begin reshaping the brain—as little as 30 minutes of vigorous movement per day can do it. This was shown in a study done by Australian scientists in which a small group of volunteers in their twenties and thirties rode exercise bicycles for 30 minutes, pedaling hard.[15] Brain scans performed afterward showed that this exercise made the volunteers' brains more plastic, meaning it was easier for their brains to remodel themselves.

In addition to increasing resilience, exercise improves the brain's ability to deal with anxiety. This was demonstrated in a 2013 study in the *Journal of Neuroscience*[16] that looked at the effects of exercise on the brains of mice. One group of laboratory mice were allowed to run on a running wheel as much as they wanted—and they wanted to run a lot, each covering about 2.5 miles per night. A second group of mice was kept in similar conditions, but without access to a running wheel, so they did not exercise.

After six weeks, all of the mice were forced to swim in cold water, a stressful experience. You would expect that this would really light up the stress and anxiety areas of their brains. But here's the fascinating thing: In the brains of the mice who exercised, brain cells in the hippocampus that dial down excitement suddenly became active. By swinging into action, these cells tamp down activity in a part of the brain—the ventral hippocampus—that plays a major role in anxiety. The exercise altered the brains of the mice in such a way that they were *less* likely than the non-exercisers to feel anxious when forced to swim in the cold water.

Exercise can also help lift the veil of depression. Many studies have shown this, with some suggesting that exercise can be just as effective as anti-depressant medications. Yet you don't have to train like an Olympian to reap results. Moderately intense exercise sessions of 30- to 45 minutes, three days a week, have been shown to significantly boost the mood and alleviate the symptoms of depression in a matter of weeks.[17]

If Exercise Is So Good, Why Doesn't Everyone Do It?

This brings us to a really important concept in pain treatment known as *fear-avoidance,* also referred to as *the fear of re-injury.* In cases of acute pain (the kind of pain you feel when you cut your finger, for example), it's helpful to rest and protect the injured body part, then give it time to heal before putting further stress on it. But with chronic pain, rest and avoidance can actually inhibit recovery by turning an active body into a "pain body." The mind can fool you into thinking that you need to protect the injured part to prevent further damage and pain, when just the opposite is true. This means that sometimes you must override your feelings about protecting a painful area, for your own benefit.

Here's an example: Let's imagine you've sprained your right ankle. You treat it with rest, elevation, and ice, and if you have to go somewhere, you use crutches to keep weight off of it. After two weeks, the inflammation and swelling goes down and it isn't that difficult to start walking and running again. Before long, you have recovered completely.

Here's a different scenario: You stay off of your ankle for six months (rather than two weeks), then attempt to start walking and jogging again. But you find that getting back to normal is much harder, takes longer, and is more complicated. When you avoid using a body part for extended periods of time (fear avoidance), weakness sets in as well as various changes made by the rest of the body to compensate. In this case, you find that both your ankle and your leg have become quite weak and your ankle joint is very stiff. There's also pain in your left knee and lower back because you've been shifting your weight to the left side for such a long time. The upshot is that it will be hard for you to start walking normally again, and your recovery will probably take a long time.

Your entire body changes for the worse when you avoid using part of it for an extended period of time. Successful recovery will depend, in part, on your ability to quiet your mental storms and put your fear "into a box."

Breaking Past the Fear

Overcoming fear-avoidance is no small feat, but you can do it! Here are some tips to help you get started:

- *Visualize success*—Create a mental image of how you will move and the kinds of things you will be able to do upon successful recovery. Imagine yourself filled with vim and vigor. Visualize that beautiful hike through the woods or that swim in the ocean that has been eluding you. Keeping your eye on the prize will help you work through the challenges.

- *Breathe*—You'll naturally tense up and hold your breath when you're anxious. And the more you tense up, the more any activity you engage in is likely to be painful. Use your breathing exercises from Chapter 5 to help relax both mind and body.

- *Find help*—We all have difficulty recognizing our own, potentially harmful, fears. An expert physical therapist or other professional can help you see which fears are impeding your progress, and suggest exercises that you can perform safely.

- *Baby steps "rock"!*—One of the keys to overcoming fear-avoidance is to make slow but steady progress. If you want to walk without a cane, begin by doing it for just fifteen minutes a day; then build slowly from there. Every little step you take is a giant leap in terms of confidence and your recovery.

- *Love your body again*—It is easy to get frustrated or angry with your body when it hurts to move it or be touched, but embrace it and appreciate it as it is. Then work with it, from this loving place.

Sometimes, when you're getting the "pain body" up and moving again, you may feel that things are getting worse, not better. But hang in there! Positive results will come and the pain will diminish—maybe it will even disappear completely.

The Best Exercise Is . . .

Now for the big question: Which is the best kind of exercise to do? Because everyone has a unique body and a unique pain experience, it's impossible to come up with a one-size-fits-all exercise program. So the best exercise program is the one that works best for *you*.

That being said, when it comes to exercise and restoring function, there are six core principles that can benefit just about everyone in pain. Keep these in mind as you craft your own exercise program.

1. *Assemble the right team of experts to assist you.* Take advantage of the knowledge and expertise of the many movement experts that are out there: physical therapists,

occupational therapists, Pilates trainers, yoga teachers, and others trained to help you move safely and more effectively. For example, physical therapists can help identify ways in which your body is off-kilter or over-compensating in unhealthy ways. Simply by watching you walk, they can identify problems with your joints or muscles, and devise an exercise program that's right for you. However, be aware that many physical therapists and trainers have *not* been trained in dealing with chronic pain. Before working with any therapist or trainer, ask about his or her background regarding your condition. You may need to search to find the one who's a good match for you.

It's critical that you develop trust and a positive working relationship with your movement specialists. Moving and exercising the "pain body" is a confidence-building process. You are likely to be entering this process with some fear and trepidation, so find someone whose understanding goes beyond mechanics, who can tune into the person inside the "pain body." It will be well worth the effort.

And don't forget that those struggling with problems similar to yours can also be valuable members of your team. The benefits that come from exercising with others can be very powerful. Consider joining a swimming group, a walking club, or some other group that can help you stay engaged and consistent. You may also pick up some useful tips from people who have successfully faced challenges like yours.

2. *Increased core strength leads to greater function and less pain, no matter which part of your body hurts.* Every stable structure needs a solid foundation. For giant redwoods, it is a rooted trunk. For the human body, it is the stabilizing muscles found in the abdomen, pelvis, and mid- to lower back, often referred to as the body's *core.* The core supports movement, lifting, carrying, reaching, pulling, stooping, twisting, turning—you name it. So whether your pain happens to be in your knees, back,

shoulders, legs, or even your hands, strengthening your body's core must always be part of the rehabilitation process. Unfortunately, our modern sedentary lifestyle does not challenge our core muscles much. And when chronic pain sets in, we move less, and our cores get weaker. The more deconditioned the core becomes, the more painful it becomes for the "pain body" to do things, creating a vicious circle of more pain that leads to more inactivity and greater pain. Thus, if you want to remain independent and perform daily activities like putting on your shoes, preparing meals, and carrying groceries, a stable core is a must.

Strengthening a weakened core requires more than just doing crunches, which actually accomplish very little. The core is a complex constellation of muscle groups running along both the front and back of the body, not just at the front of the gut. There are many ways to approach the strengthening of the core, so you have a lot of options. Physical therapists, exercise trainers, Pilates instructors, and yoga teachers can all provide you with several "core-stabilization exercises." Remember that no matter which form of exercise you choose, your program should include some core-strengthening exercises.

3. *There is always some musculoskeletal problem that needs solving.* Almost everyone in chronic pain suffers from some kind of associated musculoskeletal imbalance and muscle pain. Certain muscles just naturally tighten up or overcompensate to "get around" a pain problem. This hard-wired defense mechanism then triggers changes in body mechanics and posture. For example, perhaps you limp, hike up one shoulder, or walk in a slightly stooped position. These protective changes may help reduce acute discomfort, but they're harmful in the long run as they create new strains and pains, generating new problems.

I often see patients with painful knees or feet who have developed significant lower back pain as well. The limping and shifting of their body weight to the non-painful side leads to muscular aches and pains in the hips and back. And if this continues for a while, the upper back and neck might also begin to knot up. It's very common for someone to start off with pain in one knee and eventually develop aches and pains that radiate throughout the body.

Another common scenario begins with an acute injury along the spine caused by improper lifting or a whiplash accident. The muscles around that part of the back or neck tighten up as a protective mechanism. This may be fine at the moment, but persistent muscle tension impedes recovery. The tension must gradually be released to allow the body to twist, turn, and bend, and the pain to recede.

To identify and release dysfunctional musculoskeletal changes, enlist the help of your physical therapist, acupuncturist, massage therapist, chiropractor, or other healers trained in the art of pain relief. Then use the stretches, exercises, and self-massage techniques you learn from them to gradually work out the kinks on your own, remodeling your "pain body" so you can move more freely and with less discomfort. Be aware that "pained" muscles do have a memory, and it can take a great deal of time, persistence, and consistent work to change that memory. A few deep-tissue massages at the spa may not be enough to create the kind of sustainable change you need for true relief.

4. *Pace yourself.* Remember that you're embarking on a life-long exercise and rehabilitation program, with goals of reducing pain and improving function, not setting records. It doesn't matter how far or fast you walk, how much weight you can lift, or how many push-ups you can do in a minute. Just get moving and keep moving.

In order to do this, you must pace yourself. In the beginning, focus on improving your endurance rather than tackling high-intensity exercises. The "pain body" is often deconditioned and needs time to build itself back up; over-taxing it will only exacerbate your pain. Realize that it's necessary to limit the duration of your sessions and take breaks. Instead of exercising for 60 solid minutes and getting wiped out, try breaking it up into three 20-minute sessions spread through the day.

Know that you may feel pain when you start a new exercise program. As a general rule, if the pain fades within a few hours after exercising, you probably did just the right amount of work. The pain is a passing response to the movement and will decrease as you build your strength, flexibility, and stability. But if the pain continues into the next day, reduce the intensity of your exercise next time. You need to slow down so your body can reach a new level of fitness at its own natural pace.

Fortunately, there are many ways of achieving your exercise goals. If one approach doesn't work or is too difficult, try something else. Your physical therapist or trainer should be able to come up with multiple exercise options—and don't hesitate to ask for new options if what you've been given isn't working for you.

5. *Embrace mind/body approaches.* The "pain body" sends a flood of pain signals, fear, and anxiety through the nervous system, and this can make you want to give up on exercising before you really get started. Fortunately, you can calm your nervous system and put it at ease through various mind/body movement strategies that also prepare your body to move in new and challenging ways.

Tai chi, a combination of martial arts training and meditation, can be very helpful to a body struggling to become more active. Many of my patients find that tai chi is a pleasant way to move their bodies while improving their balance and general sense of well-being. Studies have shown that tai chi can increase strength, flexibility, and aerobic conditioning, and also reduce falls. It does all of this through coordinated gentle movements, without inflicting the stress and strain of a typical gym workout.

One of the key elements of mind/body approaches is attention to the breath, which is coordinated with body movement. As you may remember, certain breathing patterns induce the action of the parasympathetic nervous system, making you feel more at ease. Slow, deep breathing in conjunction with movement, especially stretching, is important because it helps relax both muscles and tendons, making movement easier and safer.

Mind/body practices, including yoga, Qi Gong, Pilates, tai chi, and various forms of dance, can also help the brain focus, while stimulating the positive neuroplastic changes that reduce stress and anxiety, and diminish all types of pain problems, including back pain, pain from nerve damage, and fibromyalgia. Mind/body classes are available just about everywhere. And besides being relaxing, they can be fun!

6. *Walking works.* While it may not be a particularly high-tech or exciting activity, walking is one of the best exercises available. We were created to be "walking machines," and our strength, balance, overall health, and sense of well-being improve when we walk. Walking, an excellent form of aerobic exercise, has also been shown to boost gray matter in key areas of the brain.

   Walking is a key variable in assessing a person's quality of life. How far, how long, and how fast you can walk directly influences how active, connected, and independent you can be. This means that maximizing your ability to get around should always be a critical component of your pain management program.

   The best way to incorporate walking into your rehabilitation program is simply to do it. Walk around your house, block, neighborhood, local mall, or anywhere else that seems safe and appealing. Begin by walking only as quickly and as far as you comfortably can. After that, you can slowly begin to increase your distance and speed. When you are ready to go further, start climbing stairs to improve your aerobic condition, balance, leg strength, and core stability. For many pain patients, just going up or down one step is a great starting point. Walking, and eventually adding a little stair climbing, can jump-start your pain-relief program and keep it in motion.

Move Away from Pain!

An inactive body perpetuates pain and diminishes your mental capacity and efficiency. But an active body remodels the "pain brain," positively changing the way you think, feel, process information, and respond to stress. The more active your body becomes, the less you will hurt. It's as simple as that.

CHAPTER EIGHT

Ingest Quality

Let food be thy medicine and medicine be thy food.
—Hippocrates

The way you think, move, breathe, sleep, and manage stress greatly impacts your ability to relieve pain. And what you put *into* your body, whether it be medications, food, beverages, or supplements, is equally important. There is constant interaction between what goes on in your gut and the rest of your body and mind, and the role of the gut in fighting disease and maintaining good health simply cannot be overstated. Therefore, choosing very carefully what you introduce into your gut should be an integral part of any successful pain-relief program.

Gut Bacteria: Where It All Begins

Trillions of microbes live in your gastrointestinal tract, including up to a thousand different species of bacteria. This mass, called the *microbiome,* contains more cells than the total number of cells in your entire body! Many of these microbes have a major effect on your immunity and overall well-being. For example, some protect against illness (by eating up carcinogenic substances and other invaders), some produce certain vitamins, while others trigger chronic diseases like rheumatoid arthritis or asthma. When there is a proper balance between the helpful and unhelpful microbes in the gut, good health should reign. But when the unhelpful microbes become dominant, disease can set in.

The composition of your microbiome is completely unique, and is the result of what you ingest, your environment, genetics, stress levels, and a host of other factors. Generally, the microbiome is a fairly stable community, but it can be altered by antibiotics and other medications, poor nutrition, bacterial infections, stress, and other factors. Two-thirds of the body's immune cells are housed in the gut, and they communicate with the rest of the immune system. So when the microbiome becomes unbalanced, inflammatory cells throughout the body may be activated. This is why an upset microbiome is believed to be linked to inflammatory conditions that range from obesity and autoimmune conditions to chronic pain. And it can also negatively affect your brain, ratcheting up its perception of pain.

The Gut and the Brain Like to Chat

Data collected over the past several years confirms that gut microbes communicate with the central nervous system (CNS),[1] and this communication appears to be a two-way street. This means that the microbes affect CNS function (including brain function), and the CNS, in turn, affects the microbial composition of the gut through its actions on the gastrointestinal tract.[2] Changes in the gut microflora can directly affect brain activity, while messages coming from the brain can disrupt the microflora. The gut and brain communicate with each other in a variety of ways, including through immune cell messengers, hormones, and nerve impulses that travel back and forth. And emerging research suggests that this gut–brain interaction has a big impact on overall health and well-being.

Chronic pain conditions known to have a strong link to the microflora composition in the gut include autoimmune disorders like rheumatoid arthritis (RA) and psoriatic arthritis. Those with RA, for example, are more likely to have the bacteria *Prevotella copri* in their intestines, perhaps due to a genetic disposition. Studies indicate that the *Prevotella copri* bacteria inhibit the action of some of the more protective strains of gut bacteria, which may contribute to the onset or continuance of rheumatoid arthritis.

Conversely, activity in the brain can directly alter the microflora in the gut. For example, studies show that when animals are put into stressful social situations, the composition of their gut microflora can change significantly. The stress response, activated by the brain, leads to a chain of events that includes the release of inflammatory mediators. These substances directly alter what is happening in the gut lining, and cause disruptions in the balance of the gut flora. The altered gut flora, in turn, spur the production of even more inflammatory mediators, creating a vicious cycle of inflammation promoted by both brain and gut.

Brain function also appears to be sensitive to fluctuations in the gut microbiota. Studies have found links between changes in certain gut bacteria concentrations and levels of depression, fatigue, anxiety, and perceived abdominal pain. A host of other diseases is also being looked at for links to the gut microbiota, including autism, multiple sclerosis, and obesity.

The take-home message is this: When you make decisions about what to put into your body, opt for choices that help create an optimal gut microbiome, one that will provide the best possible feedback to the ever-changing neuroplastic brain. (More on this later.)

Attack of the Glial Cells

Once the chemicals you've put into your body make it past your intestines and liver, they are off to the races, with many of them able to penetrate the blood–brain barrier and get into your central nervous system. Ideally, you want your ingestibles to reduce levels of irritating inflammatory mediators, nurture your mind, and help soothe your aching body. But if you are like millions of other Americans, you may be filling up on substances that are doing just the opposite.

In particular, I'm talking about ingesting things that may be overactivating our old friends the *glial cells*. As we discussed in Chapter 2, glial cells not only play an important supportive and nurturing role for nerves in the brain, they also play a prominent part in the genesis of chronic pain within the central nervous system. Glial cells are important to the creation of specific neuroplastic changes made by nerves within the brain. When they become over-activated by the wrong messengers, they "fan the flames" that perpetuate the pain by releasing highly pro-inflammatory, toxic mediators around the nerves throughout the "pain brain."

Once the glial cells become over-activated by factors like injury, inflammation, and stress, the inflammatory substances that are released can intensify and maintain your pain. Depending upon the type of glial cell, over-activation can cause or contribute to a string of chronic diseases, including ALS, rheumatoid arthritis, asthma, the perpetuation of obesity, and complications secondary to obesity such as diabetes.

Many things can contribute to the over-activation and over-growth of glial cells which, in turn, switch on the "pain brain." The major culprits are:

- Opioid medications (the very pills you may be taking to quell your pain)
- An imbalanced gut microbiome
- A diet high in pro-inflammatory foods
- Obesity

The good news is that you can ward off the over-activation of the glial cells, lessen inflammation, and decrease your pain simply by controlling what you put into your body.

But first, let's take a brief look at how each of the factors listed above may be increasing your pain experience.

Opioids: Painkillers That *Increase* the Hurt

It's not just the foods you eat that can create conditions that encourage pain. You also ingest medicines, which can be troublesome in their own ways.

Few topics in medicine these days garner more attention and stronger emotional reactions than opioid or narcotic-based painkillers. A surge in the prescribing of opioids (morphine, oxycodone, hydrocodone, hydromorphone, fentanyl, and methadone) seemed to take off in 2001 after Congress and President Bill Clinton announced that the new decade was the "Decade of Pain Control and Research." Prescription painkillers containing compounds like hydrocodone, oxycodone, and morphine quickly became the mainstay treatment for patients with complicated chronic pain problems. The assumption was that since opioid compounds provided the most powerful and effective relief of acute pain associated with tissue damage, they should also work for the chronic debilitating pain associated with arthritis, back pain, nerve pain, and fibromyalgia.

Today, Americans consume 80 percent of the world's opioids (including 99 percent of the world's hydrocodone), although we account for less than 5 percent of the total population. Yet since these medications have become widely available, we've seen a rise in the number of Americans who are disabled and suffering from regular daily pain. Clearly, the pharmaceutical industry has *not* solved America's pain crisis.

Many people are calling for the tightening of prescribing habits in order to curb the steep rise in accidental overdose deaths, while others warn that we should not punish "legitimate" patients who "deserve" access to opioids. (Shouldn't everyone in pain be considered a "legitimate" patient, for heaven's sake?) But once you filter out all of the "noise," you'll see that opioids are not improving the lives of those in chronic pain.

There are no well-designed scientific studies that show that long-term use of opioids produces positive results in chronic pain patients, including the relief of pain, improved quality of life, or better functionality. Or that they help improve mood or increase the feeling of well-being. In fact, it's just the opposite: Many studies have found much higher levels of concurrent emotional distress, including depression, suicidal ideation, and anxiety, in those taking opioids, which may mean their overdependence on pain pills is preventing them from addressing critical components of the chronic pain experience. So what seemed like a good idea when the "Decade of Pain" was launched has simply not panned out.

Let me be clear: I am not biased against any particular mode of treatment, and my intent is not to take anything valuable away from patients. In fact, at one time I was part of a medical community that supported the widespread use of the strongest pain medications ever known. My aim, instead, is to tell you the truth as we know it today, so you can focus on better (hopefully much better) alternatives to pain relief.

So why aren't opioids as effective for chronic pain as they are for acute pain? It appears that much of the problem lies in the way opioids interact with the glial cells. As you know, trauma, stress, and tissue injury can over-activate the glial cells and produce a panicked "pain brain," and opioids appear to affect the glial cells in a similar way.

Research has now shown that opioids such as morphine stimulate the glial cells to release excitatory messengers, which creates an inflammatory state around the nerve cells closely resembling what is seen in chronic nerve pain. This excitation of the glial cells may play a prominent role in the transformation of an acutely activated "pain brain" into the more devastating chronic "pain brain." Thus, the very medication used to lessen the pain experience, or eliminate it altogether, actually does the *opposite* over time. Flooding the nervous system with opioids simply programs the "pain brain" to stay in play longer.

Even more concerning is a phenomenon known as *opioid-induced hyperalgesia* (OIH). Hyperalgesia is the development of increased sensitivity to pain; in other words, everything suddenly hurts more than it did before. OIH is believed to be the result of neuroplastic changes throughout the nervous system. I call it the "pain pill paradox" because OIH patients actually feel *more* pain after taking opioids for an extended period of time than they did before they started.

If you have been on opioid painkillers for a while, it may be worth taking a quick inventory of how you are reacting to pain these days. Are you more sensitive than you used to be to every little bump in the road when riding in a car? When undergoing medical procedures, does it take longer for you to get numbed or sedated than it used to? Do you find yourself needing higher and higher dosages of pain medication to produce the same effect? If so, the opioid pain medications you have been taking may very well be part of the problem.

An Imbalanced Gut Microbiome

A healthy gut microbiome protects the intestines against the overgrowth of pathogens ("bad bacteria") and other harmful microorganisms. It does this by using "good bacteria" to compete for limited nutrients and "switch on" the body's immune responses when necessary.

It would be nice if we all had a healthy gut microbiome, but many of us do not. And when the balance between the "good bacteria" and the "bad bacteria" is upended, infection and inflammatory disease can result. Imbalances in the intestinal microbiota are often seen in those suffering from inflammatory bowel disease, asthma, and obesity, all of which are inflammation-related disorders. Disruptions in the microbiota can also have a direct impact on mood and well-being, causing negative changes in levels of depression, anxiety, and cognitive activity—all common problems seen with chronic pain.

Several factors can disrupt the microbiota, including

- Diets heavy in animal protein and saturated fat (especially red meat and cheese
- Opioids like morphine, which can transform the bacteria *P. aeruginosa*, normally a harmless bacteria living in the gut, into a virulent attacker of the host
- Antibiotic consumption, due to medical treatment or the ingestion of animals treated with antibiotics
- Exposure to daily toxins, including foods grown with chemicals or treated with preservatives and food coloring

A Diet High in Pro-Inflammatory Foods: Inflaming the Pain at the Snack Shack

What you eat can almost immediately affect your gut microflora. And it can also significantly tip the balance of inflammatory mediators circulating throughout your tissues, causing or quelling inflammation. A colleague of mine with rheumatoid arthritis noticed that her food choices impact the amount of swelling and discomfort she feels in her joints. But pro-inflammatory foods don't just affect your aching joints and muscles; they also make their way to the "pain brain" and surrounding glial cells. In fact, studies have shown that a high-fat diet increases the number and size of the glial cells[3] and contributes to the death of neurons in the hippocampus.

Certain types of fats are particularly pro-inflammatory: saturated fats and trans fats. Saturated fats, found in animal products like beef, pork, poultry, and dairy products, contain *arachidonic acid,* which aggravate tissue swelling and inflammation, leading to more pain. Trans fats, created by the hydrogenation of oils, are typically found in packaged crackers, cookies, snack foods, and deep-fried goodies like French fries. Trans fats increase the inflammatory mediators circulating in the bloodstream, and also increase the production of excessive amounts of arachidonic acid. I recommend that you avoid both saturated fats and trans fats whenever possible. Trans fats may be harder to spot. You'll need to become an avid label reader and avoid anything containing hydrogenated or partially-hydrogenated fats or oils, margarine, or vegetable shortening.

Too Few or Too Many Essential Fatty Acids

The omega-3 and omega-6 fatty acids are "essential fatty acids," which means your body can't manufacture them so they must be consumed through the diet. Each has a very specific effect on inflammation. Omega-3s, which are found in the fat of cold-water fish such as herring, mackerel, salmon, and sardines, are fundamental components of neuronal and glial cell membranes, and help decrease unnecessary inflammation.

Omega-6s, on the other hand, which are found in polyunsaturated fats such as soybean, corn, sunflower, or safflower oils, increase inflammation and oppose the effects of omega-3s. Although you need both kinds of fatty acids in your diet, you're probably getting far too many omega-6s, as the typical American diet is full of processed foods that contain polyunsaturated oils. Back in the days when we didn't rely on processed foods, the ratio of omega-6s to omega-3s was a healthy 1:1. But today, those consuming the standard American diet have ratios more like 15:1! This increasing exposure to diets with an unbalanced ratio of omega-6s to omega-3s drives up the level of inflammatory cytokines in the brain and increases the likelihood of experiencing pain.

Glycemic Load

Spikes in blood glucose levels trigger a chain of events that result in an increase in circulating inflammatory mediators. Continuing to overload the body's ability to process glucose spikes can eventually lead to insulin resistance and chronic problems like diabetes, cardiovascular disease, and obesity. This state of "insulin burnout" is stressful for the body and leads to a continual rise in inflammatory mediators and, thus, inflammation.

Beware of carbohydrates that promote a rapid rise in glucose. Foods made with refined white flour like breads, muffins, bagels, and pasta; sugary drinks; and white rice are among the worst culprits. The *glycemic index* is a way of measuring a given food's effect on blood sugar levels. The index assigns a numerical value to various foods based on how much they raise blood glucose levels; the higher the number, the higher the blood sugar spike resulting from eating that food. By avoiding the higher glycemic-index foods, you will expose your "pain body" and "pain brain" to fewer blood sugar spikes and less inflammation. Glycemic index ratings for most carbohydrate-containing foods are now readily available on the Internet.

Obesity

Obesity can make an already hurting body more painful to move and exercise. Weighing more often means hurting more: An obese patient is much more likely to experience pain in the head, neck, back, shoulders, legs, feet, and pelvis.

The problem has reached epidemic proportions in the United States, now affecting 35 percent of adults and 17 percent of our youth, and it can factor into the pain equation in a number of ways. Weight management is an important part of your pain relief plan for several reasons:

- Excessive weight increases mechanical forces on the body, adding stress to potentially sensitive areas like the knees, hips, and spinal column, as well as sore muscles.
- Extra abdominal fat produces inflammatory mediators that can further irritate the "pain brain."
- The glial cells, which are implicated in chronic pain, also play a part in several processes associated with excess weight gain, as well as the control of both appetite and metabolism. Although they are not thought to cause obesity, they appear to play a part in perpetuating it.

How do you know if you're overweight or obese? One way is to calculate your body mass index (BMI), using this formula: weight (pounds) / [(height (inches)]² x 703. In other words, divide your weight (in pounds) by your height (in inches) squared, and multiply the result by 703. For a woman who is five feet, five inches tall and weighs 165 pounds, that produces a BMI of 27.5. For adults, a BMI over 25 is generally considered overweight and 30 or above is obese.

Fortunately, you don't have to calculate your own BMI, for the Centers for Disease Control has an online Adult BMI Calculator at *www.cdc.gov/healthyweight/assessing/bmi/adult_bmi /english_bmi_calculator/bmi_calculator.html.*

Rethink What You Put in Your Gut

Your gut flora, the medications you take, and the food you eat all have the potential to inflame the "pain brain" and aggravate the "pain body." So it makes sense to rethink what you are putting in your gut each day. Although my recommendations are quite simple and not hard to implement, they will help you make the positive changes you both want and deserve for your mind and body. And it won't take long to see results: a change in eating habits can lead to changes in the gut's flora (for better or for worse) in as little as 24 hours.

Opioid-Based Painkillers: Tough Choices

If you haven't already begun taking potent opioid-based pain medications, my advice is to make a concerted effort to avoid them. The long-term effects on your health are negative, and they simply aren't the answer to chronic pain. Ongoing research is focusing on ways to tweak these medications to make them more efficacious and less problematic, but we just aren't there yet. And I have found that the less my patients focus on medications, the more successful they are at using alternative methods to control their pain and manage flare-ups.

However, if you are already on opioid-containing painkillers, you have some soul-searching to do. Letting go of them can be anxiety inducing, and you may wonder how you'll be able to manage the pain without them. Yet at the end of the day, you should ask yourself this question: "Do I plan on taking these medications for the rest of my life?" Before you answer, think about how your pain medications have changed your life, in both positive and negative ways. How effective have they been in helping you function and interact with the world? Which side effects have they caused, and are you prepared to live with them over the long haul? It will help to talk to your family, trusted friends, and doctors. They often see changes in you that you may not be aware of.

If you decide that you would like to get off of opioid painkillers, it's important that you have a plan and as much support as possible. Here are some tips that can help:

- Consider enlisting the support of others, apart from your doctor, as you transition away from long-term opioid use. Those you may find helpful can include a counselor, life coach, therapist, acupuncturist (acupuncture helps with withdrawals), and/or a support group made up of those who have gone through a similar process.
- Consider the timing of your transition, taking into account things like family events and holidays. December is usually not a good month for making challenging life changes.
- Develop a plan, program, or philosophy regarding the management of your pain in the future. Giving up opioids with no Plan B probably won't work in the long run. Write down how you intend to manage your physical and emotional health, and refer back to your notes during trying times.
- Consider a buprenorphine-containing medication regimen if withdrawal becomes too problematic. Buprenorphine binds tightly to the same receptors as the opioids, triggering partial activation and partial blocking. In many people, this is enough to prevent cravings for more medication.

Develop a Pain-Relief Nutrition Plan

While there isn't one specific food or eating plan that's guaranteed to lessen pain, there are important points to remember when it comes to nutrition and how you feel, inside and out. Remember, your goal is to create positive neuroplastic changes that will turn the tide in your brain, and leave you with a more vibrant body. What you choose to eat can influence this process by boosting brain activity, lowering inflammation, and shifting the balance of the flora in your intestines. It can also reduce excess weight, which can do much to alleviate your pain.

There is much to learn from the eating habits and lifestyles of people in certain cultures who traditionally live longer and experience far fewer chronic diseases. Those who live in countries bordering the Mediterranean Sea are one such example. The Mediterranean diet (which is really an eating style) got its name more than 50 years ago when researchers noticed that people living on the Greek island of Crete had long lives and low rates of heart disease and cancer, even though they consumed plenty of fat. At the time, fat was thought to be the number one cause of diet-related disease. Part of the secret of the Mediterranean diet, we've come to discover, has to do with the kind of fat they use: olive oil. A monounsaturated fat, olive oil helps lower LDL cholesterol, and contains antioxidants that prevent the buildup of plaque on artery walls and fight free-radical damage throughout the body.

Of course there's a lot more to the Mediterranean diet than olive oil. It emphasizes fresh fruits and vegetables, fish, whole grains, nuts, and legumes. Cheese and yogurt are included on a daily basis, as well as small amounts of poultry and eggs. And a daily glass of red wine (which is high in antioxidants) can also be added. However, red meat and saturated fat are eaten rarely, and only in small quantities.

The Mediterranean diet should be of particular interest to chronic pain patients because it helps ease the pain of inflammatory diseases (especially rheumatoid arthritis) by curbing inflammation, possibly because its high antioxidant content diminishes the pro-inflammatory effects of glial cells. New research also suggests that the Mediterranean diet counteracts the effects of aging on the brain and the boosting of gray matter—the opposite of what occurs in chronic pain: accelerated brain aging and diminished gray matter. Researchers have found that those who consume the Mediterranean diet also have lower body weights, and decreased risks of developing dementia, depression, heart disease, and cancer.

Seven Rules for Eating Mediterranean Style

The Mediterranean diet is easy to incorporate into your life, and full of delicious, satisfying foods. Just follow these seven rules.

1. *Load up on vegetables and fruits.* You can pretty much go wild in this category. Eat five to ten servings of fresh, nonstarchy vegetables and fruits every day. Studies show that eating at least seven servings of fresh fruit and vegetables each day significantly improves health and lowers mortality rates. Sadly, the average American consumes far less than this, so strive to make seven your lucky number every day.

2. *Keep servings of animal protein small.* Protein is essential for the growth and maintenance of every cell, tissue, and organ in your body. But, compared to Westerners, traditional Mediterranean societies consume much less in the way of beef, poultry, and pork, while still getting plenty of protein through plant-based sources and seafood.

3. *Eat two servings of fish per week.* Fish, especially those containing omega-3 fatty acids, can help fight inflammation. Studies show that those who consume high amounts of omega-3s have lower levels of inflammatory mediators like interleukin-6 and C-reactive protein. A four-ounce serving of fish, two to three times a week, is recommended although the Mediterranean communities with the greatest longevity eat seafood every day. The best fish sources of omega-3s are anchovies, herring, sardines, salmon, and other cold-water fish.

4. *Emphasize monounsaturated fats.* Monounsaturated fats (found in high amounts in olive oil and canola oil) can be good for your heart if they are eaten in moderation, especially if they replace the less-healthy saturated fats and trans fatty acids in your diet. Olives and avocados are also high in monounsaturated fats and can be eaten in moderation.

5. *Include nuts, seeds, and legumes.* Nuts and seeds are good sources of both healthy fats and antioxidants; they

also help keep your appetite under control. Studies have shown that people who eat nuts regularly tend to have lower body weights than those who don't, even though nuts have plenty of calories. Legumes (such as lentils, dried peas or beans, chickpeas, and peanuts) are great sources of vegetable protein and fiber, and contain important minerals like potassium, magnesium, and zinc. I like to bring a small bag of nuts to work to snack on, which helps me avoid eating less-healthy temptations.

6. *Change your dairy habits.* While dairy products are commonly seen in traditional Mediterranean diets, the types of products they consume have a few distinguishing traits. Cultured forms of milk, such yogurt or kefir, are favored, both of which help improve the gut microflora. Cow's milk is not consumed often; many of their delicious cheeses come from goat's milk or sheep's milk.

7. *Eat whole grains.* Whole grains (unrefined grains that haven't had the bran and germ removed, such as whole wheat, buckwheat, and brown rice) are high in fiber and slow the release of glucose into the blood. As a result, you'll experience fewer blood sugar spikes than you would with refined grains (white flour, white rice, white bread, and degermed cornflower), helping to keep inflammation levels lower. Whole grains also contain several antioxidants, minerals, and trace minerals not found in refined grains. Try using products like farro, bulgur, and quinoa in your cooking. An interesting note: Some studies have linked the fermenting process involved in making sourdough bread to positive changes in the gut microflora.

Weight Management

Weight gain is an unfortunate consequence for many living in pain. Chronic pain can interfere with meal preparation, grocery shopping, and regular physical activity, leading to lowered metabolism and less-than-optimal food choices. Before adopting any specific diet or weight-loss plan, talk to your primary care doctor, who can factor in all of your medical needs. And stay away from fad diets, as they rarely produce sustainable long-term weight loss.

Here are a few tips that can help you work toward reaching a healthy BMI:

- Always eat a good-size breakfast that includes some protein and fiber for blood sugar stabilization. Studies consistently show that skipping breakfast increases the likelihood of becoming obese, and that those who take in a larger percentage of their daily calories in the morning are more likely to have normal BMIs.
- Consult with a nutritionist or registered dietitian. You will receive a lot of practical information above and beyond what you'll get from a traditional medical doctor.
- Follow the rule of seven. Do your best to have at least seven helpings of a variety of fruits and vegetables every day. If you make a fruit bowl for yourself as part of your breakfast, you are already almost halfway there, even before the day gets going.
- Go nuts. Keep a supply of nuts handy for healthy snacking. There are lots of options including almonds, walnuts, pecans, pistachios, and cashews.
- Consult with an occupational therapist or physical therapist if your pain problems interfere with meal preparation. A therapist can help you make accommodations in your kitchen and/or strengthen the muscles you need to cook with greater ease.
- Put the "real" back into food. Go to local farmers' markets, buy locally produced foods, and begin to feel connected to the process of turning food into appealing, healthful meals.
- Read the fine print. Get into the habit of reading the labels on everything that comes from a package or a can. Avoid empty calories by shunning processed foods and sodas. It will be well worth your while to become a more discerning consumer.

In addition to these tips, try seasoning your food with herbs and spices instead of salt or high-sodium/high-sugar sauces. Herbs and spices are plant-based seasonings that are full of antioxidants and inflammation-fighting substances, and are naturally low in fat, sodium, and sugar. Make water or tea your "go to" drink, especially green tea, which is loaded with health-enhancing polyphenols. Always consume the freshest food you can find, grown locally if possible, and eat what's in season to increase the number and kind of nutrients you consume over the year. And make sure that meal time is a relaxing, fun, social event with family and friends. You'll lower your stress levels while increasing enjoyment of your meals and life in general.

Supplements

No supplement or miracle drug in the world can make up for unhealthy eating habits and poor lifestyle choices. And in general, there isn't much scientific support for using supplements or vitamins to manage pain. That being said, there are a few options to consider:

- **Fish oil**—Many studies have shown that fish oil can help fight pain. Fish oil contains omega-3 fatty acids, potent anti-inflammatory agents made up of a combination of two forms: EPA (eicosapentaenoic acid) and DHA (docosahexaenoic acid). To ease inflammation, daily doses of 2–3 grams of EPA and 1–2.5 grams DHA are recommended.
- **Alpha-lipoic acid**—If you are experiencing some form of nerve pain, consider alpha-lipoic acid, a very potent antioxidant that clears potentially harmful free radicals from the tissues. Alpha-lipoic acid has been used for years in Germany to treat painful neuropathies like diabetic neuropathy, and recent studies in the Netherlands have shown similar promise. Anywhere from 200–600 mg/day might be considered.
- **Vitamin D**—A deficiency in vitamin D has been linked to musculoskeletal pain. This is more commonly seen in those living at higher latitudes or those who spend too

much time indoors and get little exposure to sunlight. If you are concerned about being vitamin D deficient, ask your doctor to check your blood levels to see whether supplementation is warranted.

Ingest Quality Only

What you consume can alter your "pain brain" and pain experience. There is a strong connection between what is happening in your gut and how you feel—physically, mentally, and emotionally. So be extra vigilant when deciding what to put into your body, and choose foods and medications that support and enhance your recovery. Change is never easy, but it will be well worth the effort.

CHAPTER NINE

Recharge

A good laugh and a long sleep are the
two best cures for anything.
—Irish Proverb

Few things in life are more aggravating than not being able to sleep. And one of the most common and disturbing side effects of chronic pain is the lack of restful sleep. Many of my patients grapple with fatigue and burnout as their sleepless nights begin to stack up. Desperate, they often search for a "magic pill," hoping it will provide them with some bona fide shut-eye. Unfortunately, it's not the path to better sleep, at least not in the long run.

Fortunately, there are some genuinely helpful ways to refresh, recharge, and achieve a deep slumber, all of which will be discussed in this chapter. We'll also explore the important links that exist between sleep and pain, stress, mood, medications, and food.

Sleepless in Seattle, Kansas City, Knoxville, Springfield . . .

During those hours of physical and mental rest we refer to as "sleep," the brain and body repair and restore themselves. Various hormones are released, brain activity slows, body tissues grow and repair themselves, and blood pressure falls. Sleep also bolsters the immune system and helps it remain strong. It is so crucial to physical and emotional well-being that depriving prisoners of sleep has been used as a form of torture, and laboratory animals forced to stay awake for too long will die.

Pain is the number one cause of insomnia, with some 65 percent of chronic pain patients experiencing difficulty falling asleep and staying asleep, and losing an average of 42 minutes of sleep per night to pain, according to the 2015 Sleep in America Poll. But did you know that the reverse is also true: that a lack of sleep can increase your pain levels? New results from the Tromso 6 Study, a large-scale Norwegian health study, showed that people who have difficulty sleeping are more sensitive to pain.[1] In brief, study participants were separated into those who had insomnia and those who did not, and asked to thrust their hands into water that was so cold it was painful. Those with insomnia were, on average, likely to pull their hands out sooner than those who slept well, indicating that they had increased pain sensitivity. And the more severe or frequent their insomnia, the less able they were to tolerate the pain.

The most striking finding was that those who had insomnia coupled with chronic pain were more than twice as likely to yank their hands out of the cold water early, compared to those who were healthy and slept well. This suggests that chronic pain and insomnia are "synergistic miseries," each making the other worse.

Most people are well aware of the benefits of getting a good night's sleep on a regular basis: better mood and memory, improved weight control, a more powerful immune system, a better sex life, and better health overall.[2] And now we know that there's another important benefit: more sleep equals less pain. This phenomenon is apparent even in healthy people. In a recent study,[3] healthy volunteers—who did not suffer from pain but complained of being sleepy during the day—were assigned to two groups. One group was to stay in bed for 10 hours per night, while the other would continue with their regular sleep schedules.

Members of the "10 hour" group ended up sleeping 8.9 hours per night, compared to 7.1 hours for those in the other group. The extra sleep functioned as a pain killer: After just four nights, members of the "10 hour" group could hold a finger next to a heat source for a longer period of time than they could when the study began—and longer than those who did *not* get the extra sack time. More sleep provided increased resistance to painful stimulation.

We certainly need more research, but a strong connection seems to exist between a lack of restful sleep and increased feelings of pain. We don't know exactly why, but fatigue seems to reset our sensitivity to pain, increasing it and making everything hurt more.

A lack of sleep also alters the emotional state, triggering mood swings, irritability, and anxiety. And studies have shown that prolonged insomnia is strongly linked to clinical depression.[4] The pain sensitivity, anxiety and depression negatively affected by sleep are major parts of the pain equation:

$$\text{sensory} + \text{affective} + \text{cognitive-evaluative}$$
$$\div \text{ your unique body and brain}$$
$$= \text{your unique experience of chronic pain}$$

The increased sensitivity to pain caused by fatigue is part of the "sensory" element; the mood swings tie into the "affective" component of the equation. And the resulting feelings of exhaustion and burnout impact how the pain is interpreted and perceived, the "cognitive-evaluative" element. In sum, the negative effects of poor sleep fit right into the equation, ramping up your pain.

The Sleeping Brain Is a Plastic Brain

Sleep is a mysterious phenomenon; we're only just beginning to understand why it was programmed into human and animal DNA so many millions of years ago. Some have speculated that we sleep because we need to conserve energy, or because the body restores itself better when we are in a state of near unconsciousness. New research is pointing to another reason, which may turn out to be the reason that pain patients really need to sleep well. Sleep is necessary for brain plasticity, and the brain reshapes itself best during sleep, when there are fewer activities to attend to and fewer distractions. We haven't yet discovered all the ways that sleep facilitates neuroplasticity, but we do know that the brain is very active during sleep, and that sleep is necessary for consolidation of new learning and memory, tasks which require creating new brain pathways. We've also learned that sleep influences certain genes and proteins that help create new brain tissue.[5] And areas of the brain involved with storing new information, such as the hippocampus, use sleep time to expand and adapt their circuits to improve learning.

Beware the Sleeping Pills

More than 70 million Americans, including tens of millions of chronic pain patients, suffer from insomnia—a huge number of potential customers for pharmaceutical companies, and they haven't hesitated to produce one sleeping pill after another, promoting the idea that these pills are simple solutions to insomnia. Doctors, in turn, write some nine million prescriptions for sleeping pills every year, and if they truly were the solution to insomnia, we'd be one very well-rested country. But these medicines are not meant for extended use and should never be considered cures for long-term insomnia. For one thing, the sleep they produce is not as high quality as natural sleep, especially in the long run. And the pills themselves have side effects, sometimes scary ones, including lapses in memory, daytime drowsiness, balance problems, and more. You might even develop parasomnia, which means sleepwalking or engaging in activities without being aware of what you're doing. People in the grips of parasomnia have been known to eat, have sex, drive cars, and talk with people on the phone while they are still asleep.

But even more alarming is the mounting evidence suggesting the use of sleeping pills is linked to a shorter life expectancy and greater risk of developing cancer. A number of studies have looked at the link between hypnotic sleeping pills, such as Ambien, Lunesta, and Halcion, and an increased risk of death and/or cancer. A 2012 study[6] looked at over 10,000 people suffering from a variety of ailments who used prescribed sleeping pills, and compared them to over 23,000 people who did not. The two groups were followed for an average of 2.5 years, and the risk of dying for each was calculated.

The results were shocking: The risk of dying was 3.6 times higher in those prescribed eighteen doses of sleeping pills per year—just eighteen doses! That's the equivalent of popping a sleeping pill just once or twice per month. And the higher the rate of usage, the higher the risk of dying. Among those taking 132 doses or more per year, the risk of death increased more than 5 times, prompting some researchers to label sleeping pills more dangerous than smoking!

As for cancer, the same study found an increased risk of developing cancer of the lung, colon, prostate, and esophagus, as well as lymphoma, in those using the largest amounts of sleeping pills. The researchers concluded that, "Excess mortality is associated with hypnotic use, and that the increased mortality could not be explained by the health status of the participants before they began taking the sleeping pills, or the diseases they had."

We still have a lot to learn about the effects of sleeping pills, but this much is clear: They don't provide nearly as much benefit as we have been led to believe, and they are more dangerous than most of us realize. That's why I urge my patients to use them sparingly, if at all, and immediately start developing healthier strategies for getting a good night's sleep.

Tips for Getting the ZZZs

There has been a noticeable shift in American sleep cycles over the last century: We sleep less than our grandparents did. According to a 2013 Gallup Poll, we sleep an average of 6.8 hours per night, with 40 percent of Americans getting less than the recommended 7 hours of sleep per night. This is in sharp contrast to polling results from 1942, when Americans averaged closer to 8 hours of sleep and 80 percent reported getting at least 7 hours of shut-eye per night. Why the change?

It seems that our biological clocks have been altered by certain lifestyle changes. One change is that both children and adults spend a lot more time indoors during the day than they did 50 or a hundred years ago. Kids and teens are now more likely to stay inside and play computer games or use technology to communicate with each other than to go outside and play. Meanwhile, many adults are putting in long hours inside enclosed work spaces, as opposed to working outside, perhaps on a farm. Being exposed to midday sunlight outdoors is a key factor in setting our biological clocks for sleep at night. But how many of us spend even a few hours outside each day anymore?

Then there is the massive onslaught of information and communication that comes our way at all hours of the day and night, thanks to new technology. There are now an awful lot of distractions— smartphones, tablets, computers, fitness tracking bands, televisions, you name it—competing for your headspace at a time when you could be unwinding or falling fast asleep. We no longer go home at the end of the day to relax and tune out the world. Instead, many of us put in a few more hours of work at home, where we check e-mails or respond to social media activity. How can you push past all of this to get a good night's sleep? And do so without resorting to sleeping pills?

Start by creating the best-possible environment for sleep, a concept called sleep hygiene. The general idea is to create the conditions that tell your body it's time to cool down, slow certain internal activities, and otherwise prepare for sleep. Here are some tips for doing so:

- *Make "calm" the theme of your bedroom.* Try to remove as much noise and light as possible from your sleeping area. Dim the lights and bring down the room temperature ahead of time. Keep televisions, phones, and all other electronic gadgets away from your sleep space. It's much easier to fall asleep in a quiet, cool room.

- *Go outside during the day.* Exposure to sunlight during the day helps keep the body's natural circadian rhythms aligned with the rising and setting of the sun. Exposure to bright light triggers the production of the neurotransmitter serotonin, which makes you feel energetic, alert, and happy. Late in the day, serotonin is converted into melatonin, which helps you feel drowsy and ready for sleep. Producing good amounts of serotonin during the day ensures there will be sufficient melatonin at night to help you fall asleep.

- *Make time for movement.* Exercise is an excellent antidote to stress and promotes longer and deeper sleep. But
  be sure to finish exercising at least three hours before
  going to bed, as movement can rev up certain hormones,
  as well as body temperature, making it difficult to get
  into sleep mode.
- *Shun caffeine after noon.* Caffeine is a stimulant that can
  rev up the body and make it difficult to sleep. To make
  sure that it's cleared from your system by bedtime, stop
  consuming foods and beverages containing caffeine by
  noon. These include coffee, black tea, green tea, soda,
  chocolate, and cocoa, to name a few. Also, be aware that
  medications, especially headache remedies, sometimes
  contain caffeine.
- *Don't chow down late at night.* It takes a lot of energy
  for your body to digest food, especially fats and proteins. And all of this energetic activity raises the body
  temperature, the opposite of what you want when you're
  getting ready to sleep. When your body temperature
  rises (as it does in the morning), it's a signal that it's time
  to wake up. So be sure to stop eating two or three hours
  before bedtime. It's also a good idea to stop drinking
  anything, even water, so you don't have to wake up at
  night multiple times to go to the bathroom.
- *Don't drink alcohol before bedtime.* Avoid the temptation to use alcohol as a sleep aid. Alcohol has a sedating
  effect, but it disrupts normal sleep cycles and leads to
  poor-quality sleep. You'll wake up feeling tired and dull
  the next morning.
- *Wind down well before bedtime.* Don't wait until you're
  actually in bed to try to quiet your mind and body in
  preparation for sleep. Start slowing down at least an
  hour before your head hits the pillow. Switch off computers, cell phones, television, and other distractions.
  Finish up any preparations for the next day. Turn off
  unnecessary lights, and dim others. This is an excellent
  time to do relaxation exercises or meditate.

- *Set a sleep schedule, and stick to it.* Go to bed and wake up at the same time every day, even on the weekends. Creating this routine will help set your biological clock and optimize your chances of getting sufficient sleep every night. It can also eliminate "Sunday night insomnia," the inability to fall asleep on Sunday after a weekend of sleeping in. You may find that following a regular sleep schedule means you're the first one up on weekends. If so, great! You've got some quiet, uninterrupted time for yourself.
- *Remember that bed is for sleep and sex only.* A lot of people turn their beds into a combination desk/entertainment center, where they do their bills, watch television, chat on the cell phone, and so on. But turning your bed into a beehive of activity is the opposite of creating a calming environment for rest and renewal. Limit your activities in bed to sleep and love-making. Then your mind will associate your bed only with rest and pleasure.

If You Do Wake Up At Night . . .

When you wake up in the middle of the night and can't get back to sleep, it's tempting to reach for a sleeping pill or start worrying about your aches and pains. A better idea is to do some of the breathing exercises designed to quiet the mind: listening to the sound of your breath and feeling your belly move up and down as your diaphragm expands and contracts. Inhale slowly and deeply; then exhale slowly. You can also try holding your inhalation for a count of four or five.

Like everyone else, I'm sometimes too wound up to get a full night's sleep. When I find myself staring at the ceiling in the middle of the night, a special gratitude exercise seems to help me nod off in no time. I think about all the things I'm grateful for, like my family, friends, patients, or something special that happened to me that day. Then a sense of calm rapidly washes over me, and I can usually ease back to sleep in a matter of moments.

If you're not able to get back to sleep within 30 minutes or so, it's best to get out of bed. Otherwise you'll get frustrated and start to associate your bed and the middle of the night with trouble. So get up and go to another room, where you can read, fold laundry, or engage in some other relaxing or mindless activity. You might also meditate or do some relaxing yoga poses—but nothing strenuous. What you do isn't as important as what you think, so keep reminding yourself that it's perfectly natural to have trouble sleeping, especially when you're in pain. One bad night isn't the end of the world. You can redouble your efforts to get sunlight and exercise tomorrow. And if you continue to practice good sleep hygiene, you'll have an easier time of it tomorrow night.

Rx: CBT

If the sleep hygiene habits I described above don't help you enjoy the restful sleep you need, your next step should be to explore CBT, which stands for cognitive-behavioral therapy. An action-oriented form of therapy (as opposed to "talking therapy"), CBT zeroes in on the thoughts and behaviors that cause a problem. Once these thoughts/behaviors are identified, the patient and therapist work together to reduce or eliminate them.

The use of CBT to treat insomnia has been studied extensively, and there is now more scientific support for CBT as a tool for better sleep than any other modality. In one study,[7] published in the *Journal of the American Medical Association,* CBT, whether used alone or with medicines, reduced the amount of time it takes to fall asleep, as well as the amount of "awake time" during the night. It also improved sleep efficiency, the ratio of time spent asleep to total time spent in bed. The study found that long-term results are best when sleep medications are discontinued. In a separate paper on sleep,[8] which reviewed the results of five different studies, CBT was found to be more effective than sleeping pills and was recommended as a first-line treatment for insomnia.

When you enter into CBT therapy, you work with your therapist to develop good habits and handle other problems that may be interfering with your sleep. Sleep inhibitors that you may explore with your therapist can include family, job- or school-related stress, counterproductive habits like texting in bed, as well as food and medication use. You'll work on relaxation techniques that will quiet mind and body as you prepare for sleep, and even learn how to remain passively awake. This may sound a bit strange, but deliberately *not* trying to fall asleep can encourage sleep, for you're no longer trying to force something to happen and then worrying when it doesn't.

Unlike sleeping pills, CBT is designed to discover the reasons for your insomnia, then remove the obstacles to a good night's sleep.

The Painful Wake-Up Call

Being awakened by pain is often unavoidable. Rolling to one side or the other or just lying in one position too long can cause painful wake-ups. How you respond to this wake-up, however, will determine what happens next. Getting upset, agitated, or frustrated will simply make it that much harder to relax and go back into sleep. Try not to let that happen. Utilizing relaxation techniques at these difficult moments can help minimize the impact of the painful wake-up and lead to a much better night's rest.

CHAPTER TEN

Gain Treatment Perspective

A goal without a plan is just a wish.
—Antoine de Saint-Exupery

Gerald came to see me three months after he slipped and fell while on the job in a department store. A customer had spilled a drink only moments earlier on the concrete floor, making it slippery, and Gerald had taken a hard tumble. Luckily, he didn't break any bones, but by the time Gerald came to my office, he was hurting all over. On his pain diagram, Gerald drew "Xs" on his trunk, back, neck, and all four extremities. He also complained of pain around his right ankle, left knee, lower back, right hip, neck, and left wrist.

Gerald had initially gone to an urgent care center, where X-rays were taken of any areas that were symptomatic. The doctor told him that all the results were negative, but because he kept hurting in so many places for so long after the accident, Gerald grew increasingly worried. By the time we had our first meeting, he was wound pretty *tight and urged me to order five different MRIs—for his right ankle, left knee, lower back, neck, and left wrist—and refer him to a neurosurgeon, an orthopedist, and a podiatrist, right away.*

Gerald's situation was complex: He was symptomatic in so many different areas, the pain in each of those areas could negatively affect the others, and he was very anxious. It is challenging for a doctor to get a handle on complex presentations like Gerald's, and I can tell you that no insurance company wants to approve five MRIs and three specialist referrals right out of the gate. I needed to come up with a plan agreeable to both Gerald and his cost-conscious insurance company, one that would also lead to a successful, timely recovery.

The American health system is confusing, costly, riddled with contradictory advice, and designed to whisk patients through exams, procedures, and hospital stays as quickly as possible. That's because, in most cases, the faster the patients move through the system, the more money everyone else makes. Unfortunately, speed doesn't always equal success, especially in cases of chronic pain, which are usually layered like an onion, with problems at the physical, spiritual, and emotional levels.

Some of my patients have said that being "in the system" is like being strapped on a conveyor belt and worked on by one doctor after another, stopping only a few moments at each station before being whisked on to the next. "One doctor tweaks me here, the next one there, and I just roll on by," one patient told me.

This approach may be fine for manufacturing cars, but unfortunately you can't manufacture recovery or relief from chronic pain.

Pain Treatment—Often a Square Peg Aimed at a Round Hole

At my center, we treat chronic pain using multiple, complementary approaches, each of which has a proven track record. It's a "big picture" approach made up of many pieces assembled in a unique way for each patient. But you probably won't get such treatment through your regular doctor, HMO, or insurance company. Dance therapy, exercise classes, and lessons in reframing harmful thoughts are rarely offered during a doctor's office visit, and almost never covered by HMOs. That's why I'd like to spend a little time talking about how you can reconcile what works with what is typically covered by health plans. Please be aware that it will be up to *you* to initiate discussions with your doctor regarding your treatment and medications, and to figure out how best to spend your dollars and cents. It's a sad fact that no one operating within the traditional health system is going to help you with this.

I know it can be hard to think about such things when you're in pain. But taking the time to analyze the kinds of treatment offered by "the assembly line" can guide you away from treatments you don't need and toward the better alternatives. You can start by gaining some perspective on what the system has to offer, what you need to do for yourself, and what it may cost you out of pocket.

Separating the Wheat from the Chaff

You may be inundated with information from doctors, family members, friends, health websites, social media, and "regular" media, but be aware that much of it is unhelpful, useless, and possibly even dangerous.

What you need is solid facts about effective treatments and someone to guide you through an information/insurance/treatment maze that baffles even the experts. If you see five different doctors, there is a good chance you will get five different opinions about what to do. So how do you make sense of what you hear and read about chronic pain and its related problems? Let's begin with what you'll learn from your physician.

There's a good chance that your doctor won't have time to explain things carefully to you. And what he says may be peppered with confusing medical terms like *spondylitis* or *dystrophy*. Unfortunately, doctors speak to each other in what may sound like a foreign language, and many are not good about translating this into plain old English. And the issues are often so complex that words may not help you understand what is happening inside your brain and body.

Articles in magazines and newspapers, health segments on TV, and information presented on daytime talk shows may offer up-to-date, accurate information about your health condition, but it's often presented out of context. You might, for example, read an article about the results of a study on a new pain medicine, but one single study is not a good representation of reality. And even studies that are well designed will have a limited focus, run for a finite and usually brief period of time, and examine a small population—often a hundred people. Such studies produce helpful information, but they are just small pieces in the very complex pain puzzle.

As for the Internet, while it's a repository of potentially valuable information, it cannot be objective or come up with any kind of tailor-made "cure" for your specific predicament. Nor is it well-regulated for accuracy or authenticity. Internet search engines like Google, Bing, or Yahoo! have secret algorithms or "rules" for determining which websites appear at the top of the search list. The companies or people that run the websites focus more on appeasing the search engines so they'll gain a good position, than on providing the most relevant, helpful, and in-depth information possible. Thus, a site may or may not have great information. But you can't be sure, either way.

Community sites are growing in popularity on the Internet. People suffering from similar conditions will post messages about their symptoms and treatments and offer advice and support. Health practitioners of all kinds may also weigh in, offering their own opinions. There are pluses and minuses to these sites. On one hand, you certainly take a risk when you follow the advice of a total stranger on the web. On the other hand, you just might pick up on something valuable that your doctor hasn't thought about or told you about—something you can mention during your next appointment.

In recent years, we've seen a huge increase in the number of health-related mobile apps that can be downloaded to a smartphone. But how do you sift through all that claim to be relevant to your particular medical condition? Ask yourself: Who developed the app? What are their qualifications? What is their purpose—are they providing unbiased information, pushing a product, or what? Be aware that using apps to help manage pain is a brand new idea that has not yet been subjected to scientific study.

Then there are the social media sites, where you can interact with other people suffering from pain similar to yours. These might be helpful, but remember that any information about yourself and your condition that you disclose on social media sites—or on any community sites—will be reviewed carefully by organizations with deep pockets who hope to profit by learning about your pain. You have no privacy on the web.

Seeking out medical information about your condition is a positive thing, a sign that you are actively engaged in improving your health. But remember that the information you get from the Internet is a mixed bag, and it can be very difficult to decipher even the most accurate information. So when you find something interesting, read it carefully and consider the source. Is the information or advice coming from a physician? An herbalist? A layperson? A fellow pain sufferer? An attorney? A company that wants to sell you something? Or is there no indication at all who wrote the article or post? Identify the source; then do a little digging to see if you can discover a reason for bias. You can't always tell, but it's worth a try.

The Skinny on Studies

So far, I've been talking about health studies as if they're all the same—but they aren't. There are several different kinds of studies, each designed to uncover various kinds of information.

For example, *cohort studies* follow large groups of people over time, watching to see what happens. The researchers don't do anything; they simply observe the members of the group, then report what they find. For example, the researchers might track 10,000 people over 20 years, then look at the data and report that those who exercised more than three times a week developed less heart disease. This is very useful information, but it doesn't prove that exercise reduces the risk of heart disease. It could be that those who exercised more were healthier to begin with, or were more likely to consume healthy diets, which was what really protected them against heart disease. It's also possible that the link between more exercise and less heart disease was just a statistical coincidence.

We doctors prefer to base our treatments on *prospective, double-blind studies,* which are felt to be the "gold standard" of studies. These studies are

- *Prospective,* which means that at least two groups of people are followed over time to see how a certain treatment fares. One group receives the treatment, while the other group, called the "control group," does not. The

control group may receive a different treatment, or no
treatment at all.

- *Double-blind,* which means that neither the researchers nor the participants know which group is getting the
  treatment and which is not. For example, if the study
  required the participants to take a new medicine, everyone would take pills that looked exactly the same so
  that no one would know which participants were taking the "real thing." There are good reasons for this: If
  the researchers know which participants are getting the
  treatment, they might be tempted, consciously or sub-
  consciously, to rate their outcomes higher than deserved.
  And they might do the reverse if they know which participants are in the "control group," taking the placebo.
  Meanwhile, the participants are also "blinded" to reduce
  the influence of the placebo effect, which can cause
  improvements simply because the participants believe
  the "medicine" will make them better.

- *Randomized,* which means that participants are arbi-
  trarily assigned to receive either the treatment or something else. For example, those in the "treatment group"
  might participate in art therapy led by a trained art
  therapist, while those in the "control group" might be
  asked to sit and draw whatever they wish, or listen to
  a lecture on good health habits. By randomly assigning
  participants to treatment or control groups, no one can
  "stack the deck" by putting certain patients into a group
  more likely to produce a certain result.

Prospective, double-blind, randomized studies published in
respected medical journals carry a lot of weight. But a *meta-analysis*
is even heftier. This is a "study of studies," created when numerous studies on the same topic are combined and, using statistical
tools, create a larger study. For example, separate studies with 100
participants, 250 participants, 75 participants, and 300 participants
may be combined into a meta-analysis of 725 people. Larger studies
are considered more valid, as they're less likely to be influenced by
chance events.

When considering how much weight you should give to the results of a study, find out what kind of study it is. Cohort studies may provide useful information, but only a prospective, double-blind, randomized study puts the treatment to the test. Of course, even these studies have their limits. But ideally, many prospective, double-blind, randomized studies will come to the same conclusion, as shown by a meta-analysis that includes these studies.

Getting Through to Your Doctor

In an ideal world, you'll leave your doctor's office with a well-defined plan for managing your chronic pain. You'll have good answers to all of the questions you asked during your visit, and you'll truly understand the issues surrounding your pain. But this is unlikely to happen if your doctor is on a tight schedule. When a doctor is only allotted twelve to fifteen minutes per patient, she must rush through a list of required items before even considering anything else. And because everything must now be documented on a computer, many doctors spend much of the visit typing on a keyboard, when they should be communicating with the patient.

For patients, trying to get information from their doctors or asking about a new treatment approach can be difficult; most doctors don't let their patients talk for more than 10 to 15 seconds before they interrupt them. And most are focused on the pills and procedures they studied in medical school, which they continue to use every day.

To make the most of your time with your doctor, gear the conversation toward your goals. Discuss what you hope to accomplish through treatment. Think about the five key goals that were discussed in Chapter 4: mobility, interaction, independence, validation, and love. Write them on a piece of paper (along with any other goals you might have) and refer to it when talking to your doctor.

Then explain your biggest concerns to your doctor and why they bother you, but resist the temptation to rattle off a litany of symptoms and complaints. One of my long-time patients comes in every few months just to tell me she is worse. That's all she says, which is not very helpful to me. Naturally you need to report the things that are bothering you, but your entire visit can be eaten up by your complaints and your doctor's response, which will likely be writing prescriptions for you. In short, if you want your visits to be more meaningful and impactful, focus as much as possible on your goals.

Here are some tips for communicating more effectively with your doctors:

- *Be specific.* Focus on the real-life problems you need help with. For example, if your back hurts too much for you to prepare meals, spend some time analyzing the situation before you arrive. Break down the mechanics, tell your doctor how high your counter tops are and how heavy your pots and pans are. Physically show your doctor what happens when you engage in this activity to paint a more vivid picture that will improve your doctor's appreciation of the situation.

- *Don't be afraid.* Your doctor should make you feel that you can ask about anything that pertains to your health. If she uses a term you don't understand, ask her to explain it in layman's terms, so there are no misunderstandings. Touchy subjects like sex can be harder to bring up, but if you don't ask, she won't be able to help you. If you simply don't feel comfortable talking to your doctor, consider finding someone else.

- *Drop the agenda.* Instead of going into an appointment thinking that your doctor needs to increase your dosage of pain medication—or else!—let him know that you are struggling with your pain, and list the specific ways in which you are struggling. Then be open-minded about discussing different methods of controlling that pain; for example, trying a new way to calm down a bad bout of sciatica.

- *Be prepared.* Bring a list of questions and concerns with you to your appointment so you can go over them with your doctor. But try not to overload her with too many questions during one visit. Always begin with the most important ones, to make sure they will be addressed.

- *See the forest.* Keep the vision of recovery foremost in your mind. Getting stuck in the details can cause you and your doctor to lose sight of what you are really trying to accomplish. Periodically remind him of what the big picture looks like to you, so he doesn't lose sight of the major goal.
- *Ask the "Golden Question."* Ask your doctor if she would recommend a certain treatment or medication to her own mother or spouse, if they were suffering from your problem. Doctors should only recommend what they believe is viable for themselves and the significant people in their lives. If the answer isn't a quick and firm "yes," you'll know there is a problem.
- *Share gratitude.* Yes, you are seeing your doctor because you don't feel well and need help. But don't forget to let her know about any positives, things that the treatment has improved. For your doctor, getting a "thank you" can be priceless.
- *Be social.* Most doctors love to learn interesting things about their patients—their lives, careers, and families. We also appreciate it when you ask how we are doing and see us as human beings. I used to love my visits with a patient who told me stories about piloting planes during World War II. Creating an emotional connection with your doctor can help him understand you better.

Dollars and Sense

Being a patient in pain can be very hard on your wallet. Millions of chronic pain patients spend thousands of dollars a year on tests, treatments, medicines, and devices. And yet, if you analyze years of outcome data on interventional and surgical treatments for pain, you will be disappointed. For example, the relief offered by epidural steroid injections is usually short-lasting and often must be repeated over and over again. And back pain patients who have spinal surgery often end up with the same amount of pain as those who do *not* undergo the surgery. Today's standard treatments for chronic pain—medications, procedures, and surgeries—are not only costly, but increase the risk of needing future treatment. And, surprisingly, they lack the evidence-based scientific support to demonstrate their long-term efficacy and value.

Isn't it time to regroup and shift all of this spending to alternatives that actually help heal the "pain brain" and offer better long-term results? It's a sad state of affairs that such treatments are not covered by most types of insurance and require out-of-pocket payment. But it's vitally important that you allocate time and money to treatments that will be *transformational*—that will help you build lasting and meaningful change, actively engage in life, and become more independent. Transformational treatments will probably cost you money, but eventually there will be an end to your cash outlay. Unlike standard pain treatment, they do not have to be repeated indefinitely to remain effective.

For example, let's suppose you want to work on improving your aching back. One option is to see a pain management specialist who prescribes a state-of-the-art painkiller. You take the medication regularly and it seems to help, but only if you keep taking it. What is the end game? How long must you continue to see this doctor for medication refills? One year? Two? Maybe ten? Your out-of-pocket costs will vary depending upon your insurance coverage, but regardless of what you pay, you will still be chronically dependent on this medication and the doctor who prescribes it. This is not a transformational situation; it's more like being a hamster on a wheel.

Now suppose you take a different direction and begin working on your back pain with a Pilates instructor. After a few months of weekly sessions, your core muscles have begun to support your back better and the tight muscles around your spine have eased up and become more flexible. After investing in a dozen or so Pilates sessions, your back pain is under better control. At this point, you know enough so you can do some of the exercises and stretches on your own; this means you can cut back on your paying sessions. Your body has changed and you feel good. Now *this* is a transformational treatment!

It's frustrating that mindfulness-based stress reduction courses, tai chi classes, Pilates, art therapy, EMDR, and other modalities that make positive changes to the "pain brain" are rarely covered by insurance plans or Medicare. But what you're spending on standard treatments may also be quite hefty. And how much benefit have you received? There may be expensive copays and deductibles for medicines that haven't produced the desired results. You may have paid in part or in full for MRIs or other tests, yet they do nothing to quell your chronic pain. You've probably spent (or lost) plenty of money on things like a special bed, mattress, and/or pillow because you aren't sleeping well; vitamins and other supplements for joint inflammation; time off of work due to pain; or having to go on disability. And what about the personal things you've given up? You can't put a price tag on missing your child's recital, not being able to join a friend for a jog in the park, or not being able to walk along the beach with a loved one.

Invest your time, money, and effort on treatments that can truly reduce your pain, restore function, help you regain control over your life, and infuse you with hope so you can continue moving forward. At the end of the day, what you will really be investing in is you—in your health, your well-being, and the life you want to lead.

CHAPTER ELEVEN

It's Just a Matter of Time

We must use time as a tool, not as a couch.
—John F. Kennedy

Success is the ability to go from one failure
to another with no loss of enthusiasm.
—Winston Churchill

How do you see yourself—today, right now? How would you like to see yourself? What needs to change in your life for that to happen?

Back in Chapter 5, we talked about an art project called The Bridge, in which you draw a picture of what your life is like now on the left side of a sheet of paper, and a picture of what you want your life to look like on the right side. In between the two you draw a bridge. This bridge represents your path from who you are now to who you want to be in the months and years to come. Naturally, you must cross that bridge to reach your better, brighter future.

Do you feel stuck at the beginning of your bridge? If so, what changes do you need to make to reach the other side?

Are You Aligned With Your Vision?

If you analyze your mental image of your best future, you will likely see that it includes many of the core values we've discussed: mobility, interaction, independence, validation, and love. Are you currently on a path that will bring these core values back into your life? In other words, are your actions in alignment with your goals? If you find that you're not moving across that bridge, it's time to re-think your approach to renewal and recovery.

I've seen many people take on the role of "professional patient." They describe their typical day in terms of going to medical appointments and taking painkillers. Their lives revolve around seeking help, unable to take charge of their own situations, which puts them in a passive, dependent state. But if a pain patient needs to see a doctor every month for the rest of his life, something isn't working. I tell such patients that one of my goals is to get them to a place where they don't need me anymore. I want them to shed the "professional patient" persona and devote their time to becoming strong, healthy, independent people.

Other patients struggle with a different predicament. As breadwinners working long hours to support their families, or caregivers raising families or looking after elderly parents, they are too busy to manage their own pain. Overwhelmed by responsibilities, they never seem to find time to take care of themselves, so they remain stuck in their pain. But achieving good health doesn't just happen. Crossing the bridge takes time, commitment, and perseverance.

Time Is on Your Side

This brings us to our final concept in the book: time. Time is a key factor in your recovery. Though it takes only about 24 hours for an injured body to begin to atrophy, it can take months or even years to build it up again. But time shouldn't be a negative factor. It can become a powerful healing tool, for every moment is an opportunity to heal the "pain brain" and "pain body." Maybe only a tiny bit of healing can occur in any given moment, but over time these tiny bits add up, leading to a healthier, more viable you.

Remind yourself that every minute you spend walking, releasing pent-up emotions, quieting your mind, or doing anything else that heals the "pain brain," propels you a little further across the bridge and toward your goal. This means that every moment is precious.

Multiplying the Power of Time: Structure and Support

At my center, we offer a comprehensive structured program designed to help patients acquire the tools and master the skills that can relieve their pain and restore their lives. Patients engaged in this program put in a lot of time and hard work. They are with us six hours a day, five days a week, for six weeks—180 hours spent with me and my staff. Yet many wish they could spend even more time.

Our patients learn some great lessons from this intensive approach, one of the most important being how to structure their time. Just by coming to the clinic, they change the way they spend their time and what they focus on. Their time is structured: They exercise, meditate, work on art projects, and mentally/verbally process things that may make them feel uncomfortable. And they soon recognize the importance that structure plays in the therapeutic process. Many have been unable to work, or have been locked up in their rooms for extended periods of time, watching the days drift away. Building a daily/weekly schedule that includes healthy lifestyle habits and positive life experiences, and being accountable for following that schedule, is a powerful step toward success. Think of the typical high-powered CEO who needs to get a lot done in a day. She's always on a tight schedule, zipping from one task or appointment to the next, day after day. The energy generated by one task propels her into the next one. By the end of the day, she may have accomplished more than other people do in a week. You can use this as a model for your own pain management program: Become the CEO of your own recovery.

This doesn't mean, however, that you should just muscle through your recovery on your own without help. The patients in my program engage in all activities with other pain patients. Working with others who are fighting a similar battle, and winning that battle, is very powerful, and healing is contagious. For example, when one patient with a serious back problem starts to feel better and do more, her success instills hope and confidence in the rest of the group.

Positive social support from your peers as you work toward healing is a source of several important core values. For example, participating in a group fulfills the core value of interaction. Seeing that others are going through situations similar to yours fulfills the core value of validation. And being encouraged and supported, while offering the same to others, fulfills the core value of love.

Don't try to go it alone. Being with others supercharges your recovery.

Building a "Pain-Relief Village"

Even if you aren't able to engage in a comprehensive structured pain management program, you can easily access the healing power of being with others. And if you do attend a program, you can continue working with others once you finish.

Every day, try to spend time doing something with other people. For example, you and a friend might take a daily walk together or you might join a walking club. Perhaps you can get involved in a group hobby: knitting, playing chess, dancing, doing tai chi, listening to music, or anything else that's enjoyable and gets you out among others. Helping other people is a great way to take your mind off yourself and improve your emotional, spiritual, and physical health, especially when you're working alongside other people. Consider joining a community group or church club that sponsors charitable activities.

Connecting with others can be a process, and one that you may not feel comfortable with at first. But remember, there are a hundred million others out there dealing with pain on a daily basis, many of whom probably also feel isolated and nervous about what to do. Here are some tips to help get the ball rolling:

- *Use your doctor's office as a resource.* If there isn't a support group available in your area that interests you, talk to your doctor about volunteering to start something for the other patients in the practice. Perhaps you could post a sign-up sheet in the waiting room?

- *Therapist-led groups.* Community-based pain psychologists, for example, often hold group sessions for their clients. Mindfulness-Based Stress Reduction programs are popping up all over the country and are usually held after work. Local hospitals, universities, or medical centers may help you find available resources.
- *Social media.* You can often find local resources on the Internet and popular social networking, or create new ones.
- *Build passion.* Not everyone is looking for a crocheting group or book club that focuses on reading about health, but a lot of times folks start to really appreciate these types of pursuits once they try them. It helps to keep an open mind.
- *Avoid the culture of toxic.* It's important to find groups, clubs, and social interactions that support your positive growth and development. Too much negative energy can spoil the experience, so try to foster groups with a healthy balance between the need to process and express all the challenges wrapped around chronic pain, and the need to learn and discuss effective coping strategies and tools.

There's a healing magic that can come from working with others who understand what you are going through, in an environment where everyone feels safe, supported, and able to share. You'll find that the more you give to others, the more you'll get back in terms of empathy, knowledge, support, and love, increasing your sense of well-being and decreasing your pain. Being with others can be powerful, almost magical.

Machines and Gadgets

Most of us spend a significant amount of the day interacting with machines and gadgets, everything from smartphones, televisions, and computers, to cars, buses, and power tools. But is overuse or improper use of these machines and gadgets aggravating your pain? It may be time to change your body mechanics.

Technological conveniences are not always pain friendly, considering our bodies feel best when we allow them to move freely. Think, for example, of all the time we spend sitting slouched in chairs and hunched over our computers and other gadgets. Since the human frame was not designed to sit frozen at a keyboard for long hours, it's not surprising that we've seen a huge increase in neck, back, wrist, and hand problems in recent years. The latest malady is "text neck," injury to the neck, upper back, and shoulders caused by looking down at wireless devices for too long.

You may want to consult with a therapist or ergonomic expert who can take a careful look at how your machines and gadgets may be enhancing your pain, and what you can do about it. Sometimes it's a simple matter of raising your computer screen to the right level. Other times, more complex readjustments may be required.

Your computer chair is vitally important. A good chair should provide maximal support while keeping your body in the least stressful position. The ideal computer chair should have the following:

- Adjustable armrests to support your arms from the elbow to the wrist at a 90-degree angle to your torso. This keeps your wrists in the proper position (helping to avoid carpal tunnel syndrome) and eliminates strain on your arms and neck.
- Built-in support for your lower back, allowing you to sit up straight with your head and torso erect.
- A seat with adjustable height and angle so your feet will be flat on the floor or on a foot rest, and your thighs and shins will create a 90-degree angle.

Your computer workstation must also to conform to your body properly:

- Your desk should be on the same plane as your bent elbows when keyboarding. That is, your arms shouldn't angle upward or downward, and your wrists shouldn't bend while you work. A keyboard that sits too high can make you shrug your shoulders, and can strain your wrists. If it sits too low, your arms and wrists won't be supported properly.
- The top of your computer screen should be slightly below eye level so your head isn't angling up or down as you read.

- You should be able to read comfortably when your eyes are eighteen to 28 inches from the screen. (Since reading glasses are designed for lesser distances, you may need to get special computer glasses to keep from craning your neck to get a better look at the screen.)
- When working at the computer, be sure to change positions often. Stand, stretch, and move about as much as possible. Consider setting up timed reminders encouraging you to move around every 30 minutes or so.
- As for the phone, if you use one at your desk for more than a few minutes a day, you may do well to get a headset. Nothing can tie your neck in knots faster than holding a phone receiver with your shoulder as you type!

Of course, these are not the only ergonomic changes you can make to help ease your pain; but they give you an idea of the simple things you can do to prevent your daily routine from contributing to your pain.

Never Give Up!

Many patients have told me that they believe their situation is hopeless, so there's no point trying. This raises a few important questions: What do you believe you can do? And how do you think that belief influences what you *try* to do?

When I first met Lucas, he was really angry: He was sick and tired of being poked and prodded by one doctor after another, not one of whom had been able to help him. He was frustrated that modern medicine could not supply him with a pill or treatment that would make his dreadful sciatica disappear. After being disappointed by one doctor and one treatment after another, he considered his situation hopeless and just wanted somebody to prescribe something to knock him out. "If I can't feel good," he said, "I want to feel as little as possible."

When I told him that I really couldn't solve his problems that way, he got even angrier. He told me I was a lousy doctor for not putting an end to his suffering. Without thinking, I replied that he wasn't suffering because of his pain: the problem was his *attitude* about his pain. Yikes! Did I really say that to a brand-new, already upset patient? I really thought I blew it, but his demeanor suddenly lightened up dramatically. "Tell me more," he said.

We talked about how he had been stuck in a rut by his attitude and frustrations, and how he was hampering his search for relief. Lucas began to share his experiences of fighting in Vietnam. He had overcome so much tragedy in his life; but he realized that, this time, he was standing in his own way. He walked out of the office that day feeling liberated and believing that maybe he could conquer his pain.

Psychologists have a term to describe a person's belief in his ability to do something: *self-efficacy*. When you have self-efficacy you believe that you *can* accomplish a task, whether it's exercising regularly, giving up cigarettes, losing weight, improving your grades in school, mastering stress management techniques, reading the works of the Great Masters—or even turning a "pain brain" into a healthy brain.

I often work with patients who depend on a cane to get around when they first come to my office. In some cases, my rehabilitation team and I believe we can help a patient learn to walk again without the cane. But *my* belief that a person can develop enough balance, strength, and pain control to gradually give up the cane is not enough. That person must also believe it.

The concept of self-efficacy was developed by psychologist Albert Bandura in the 1970s. Since then, a great deal of research has validated the idea, and demonstrated that having self-efficacy, or confidence in your ability to succeed, has a tremendous impact on your thoughts and actions. People with a strong sense of self-efficacy see problems as challenges, and bounce back from setbacks. They learn from their defeats and believe they can regain control of certain circumstances. Those with a weak sense of self-efficacy, on the other hand, are more likely to avoid dealing with the problem all together, and will interpret any setback as proof that they can't succeed and are not in control of their circumstances. For them, there's simply no point in trying.

Fortunately, there are ways to build self-efficacy, even if you don't have much at the moment. Here are a few ideas:

- *Build a record of small successes.* If walking is difficult for you, walk for just two minutes today, or even just two steps. Then take three steps tomorrow, or walk for three whole minutes. In a few weeks, you'll look back and be proud of what you've done—and believe you can do more.

- *Think of your past successes.* In your work, hobbies, interpersonal relationships, or intellectual pursuits, you've been the "champ" many times. Although these activities may not be related to your chronic pain, they are directly related to *you*. You are the one who over-came the hurdles, put your nose to the grindstone, devised a new approach that led to success, and so on. You are capable of doing great things. And you can apply your talent and your willpower to today's hurdle, as well.

- *Give and get support.* When you help others, you create a powerful new mindset. You're no longer a helpless vic-tim of circumstances; you're a doer and a believer. You believe that it is possible for the person you're helping to move forward and you believe that you are strong/wise/compassionate enough to help him do so. If it's possible for someone else to succeed, and if you are strong/wise/compassionate enough to help, you can succeed, too. Asking for support is just as empowering, for it means that you believe your goal is possible. Simply believing it is possible makes it more probable that you will accom-plish it—if not today, then in the near future.

- *Forgive your stumbles.* If you're a human being, you're going to stumble and occasionally fall flat on your face. That's just a part of life. When you stumble, ask yourself why, learn the lessons, make any necessary adjustments to your thoughts or actions, and just start moving ahead again.

- *Visualize future successes.* Start to imagine what it will be like on the other side of the bridge. See yourself moving about unencumbered, see yourself happy, see yourself at work and at play, see yourself having fun with your friends and family, and see yourself helping others. Just visualizing yourself doing all that you desire will bring you closer to achieving it.

Building your self-efficacy is like putting on glasses that let you see farther "across your bridge," into the happy future you've created. The more you believe you can cross that bridge, the easier each step will be.

Xs and Os: Draw the Winning Game Plan

Get a piece of paper and draw a line down the middle, from top to bottom. On the left side, write down what you do on a typical day, including how much you walk, lie down, and sit; what you eat; the chores you do around the house; and when you sleep. Are the ways you spend your time and energy in line with your goals—your vision of life on the other side of the bridge?

Look carefully at your daily schedule. Are there time periods or tasks you can change? Are there minutes here and there you can devote to exercise, quieting your mind, interacting with others, helping others, or otherwise healing your "pain brain?"

Now create another daily schedule, on the right side of the paper, one that will better help you reach your goals and attain your core values. You don't have to pack your day full of healing activities; if you just get a few in, that's a great start. For example, the new schedule might include time for exercise, time to take breaks from the computer, time for meditation and prayer, and time to do something for others. Just by thinking through these changes, you'll be on your way to a better life.

Casino Royale

I often tell my patients that the world we live in is like a casino. What do you see when you first enter? Lots of bright lights with constant noise and stimulation, but no doors or windows. Why? Because that is how they get your money; the sensory overload keeps you from leaving. Casinos don't want you to have a focus or a direction. The more overwhelmed you are by blinking lights and ringing bells, the more likely you are to keep on gambling without thinking about your losses.

Living in our modern society can be very much like being trapped in a casino. We are bombarded by stimulation and sensory overload from our machines and gadgets, distracting us with calls, texts, e-mails, advertisements, videos, shows, messages—you name it. It's become easier and easier to stop focusing on our goals and lose our way. But instead of losing money in a slot machine, we lose something much more valuable: time. And for chronic pain patients, this is truly a loss because time is a critical element in remodeling and reshaping the "pain brain" and revitalizing the "pain body." Pain relief requires structure, discipline, and regularity. It requires a plan. If you just allow life to sweep you along, you probably won't find the time to address all of the elements of a successful pain management program. So make time for quiet and stillness in your life, time when you can filter out all the noise and keep yourself centered on what is important. Then devise a structure that you can live with and begin your journey across the bridge. You can do it! But it will take time, focus, and persistence.

In the words of Steve Jobs, "Time is the most precious resource we all have." Using your time wisely will give you the power to help yourself and help others.

Two Steps Forward, One Step Back

The race is not always to the swift,
but to those who keep on running.

—Anonymous

Pain relief is often as much a "mind game" as a physical one. Your pain plays tricks on you, distorting how you see yourself, and changing what you think is possible. One of its clever ploys is to take the words you hear and twist them, increasing the harmful chatter inside your mind. For example, when you hear the word "degenerated," you can start to think "impossible to overcome." And when you hear words like "herniated" or "ruptured," you might become convinced that your situation will never improve until it gets *"fixed."*

An ironic twist shook my world shortly after I started writing this book. It began when I tweaked my lower back while working out. After a few weeks I was able to resume my regular exercise routine, but then my back locked up again. This time, the pain in my lower back was so intense I had a hard time bending or moving. This second episode lasted for several weeks before everything finally calmed down again—or so I thought.

Feeling better, I decided to go for a bike ride one Saturday morning. But once I got off my bike, I began to feel a pounding sensation in my left buttock. "Must be a muscle spasm," I thought, although I had never felt one like that before. The next night, I suddenly felt a burst of burning electrical pain shoot down my left leg. It was so painful that I couldn't find a single comfortable position, and all I could do was pace back and forth. The pain grew even more intense over the next several days, to the point where it felt like somebody had poured lighter fluid down the back of my leg and set it on fire.

Within a matter of days, I could no longer sit, drive, or sleep, and going to the bathroom had become a real challenge. I lost feeling in my left leg and foot, my leg began to atrophy, and before I knew it, I had lost about four pounds worth of muscle in that leg. An MRI of my lumbar spine showed I had a herniated disc and had extruded a large piece of disc material. The extruded fragment had pinned one of my nerve roots against the bone around my spine. "Holy crap!" I thought when I saw it.

For the next several weeks, I was forced to do everything standing up; the nerve was trapped and could not tolerate being stretched to the point where I could get into a sitting position, not even for a second. This meant that I had to maintain a standing position all day while seeing my patients, and my wife had to drive me to and from work while I lay on my stomach on the back seat. At noon, I would crash on my office floor before starting my afternoon appointments. I ate all of my meals standing up, placing a cardboard box on a table so the plate was at chest level. But the nights were the worst. I could only stand being in bed for a few hours at a time before the electrical pain in my leg became unbearable. Then I'd get up and pace around the house like a caged animal for at least an hour, until the pain finally settled down. Needless to say, I was sleep deprived for weeks.

During this time, a number of dramatic changes took place in my body. My walking capacity dwindled to about two blocks, and I went from being a pretty fit, middle-aged man to being unable to put on my own shoes and socks. My blood pressure went through the roof. And a few months into my recovery, I came down with one of the worst flus that I have ever experienced. Bedridden, coughing, retching, and vomiting, I finally reached my breaking point. I broke down crying when I told my wife, "I can't do this anymore!"

I frequently felt apprehensive, especially when well-meaning people said things like "You need to have surgery or you'll never get better." While Dr. Abaci, the physician, never believed this was the case, Peter Abaci, the vulnerable patient, felt angst whenever he heard anything even slightly discouraging. Another wave of fear washed over me whenever I saw patients with problems similar to mine who continued to struggle with basic daily activities like putting on their shoes, going to the bathroom, and being intimate with their partners. What was *my* life going to be like? Was I going to have permanent nerve damage? What would I do if the feeling and strength did not come back to my left leg and foot? After all the years I'd spent helping others overcome such problems, I was scared to death about my own fate.

Within the first week, I lost the ability to raise my left heel when standing. And right about that time, I saw a patient who had the same deficit. She told me her orthopedist said that this symptom meant she needed back surgery. Another wave of panic slammed into me. Would my left leg never work properly if I didn't rush to the operating room? When excruciating pain is continually shooting down your leg, it's tempting to accept just about any kind of treatment just to make the pain go away.

Yet, all throughout this terrible time, another inner voice was telling me to hang tough and work through whatever came my way, one step at a time. In preparation for writing this book, I had been studying the latest research on topics like spine surgery, opioids, meditation, and resiliency. I began to reflect on the studies I had read, the patients I had treated, and ways I had overcome previous difficulties in my life. And I came up with one irrefutable conclusion: There was *hope*.

When I tell people about my own injury, they are always curious about the methods and treatments I chose to help myself heal. Surely, a pain doctor must have some kind of magic up his sleeve to save his own skin! So let me share with you the battle strategy I adopted.

One of my main goals was to do whatever I could to aid my body's natural healing methods. Research on large extruded discs has shown that, over a period of months, immune cells move in to clean out the disc material, and this became a focal point of my strategy. I didn't want to put anything in my body that could interfere with this immune cell clean-up job. That meant avoiding painkillers, cortisone shots, and surgery, no matter how much I was hurting.

Instead, I opted for acupuncture, hoping it would enhance my immune response by improving circulation to the area, boosting my qi, and who knows what else. The first session left me feeling better for only a few hours, but I decided to try again. The second session seemed to help for about three days, and that was enough to keep me going back once a week for several weeks. My body responded favorably to these treatments, and that made my hope grow brighter.

Besides aiding the healing process, I needed a plan to help my body recover. There were crazy things happening: a constant cramp in my left calf, a nonstop twitching in my left buttock, knots all over my back, numbness in my foot, and skin sensitivity in spots on my left leg. I went to a physical therapist who specialized in Pilates, since that had worked well for me when I'd had a knee injury. She worked with me on Saturdays, and gave me exercises to do during the week. This painstaking restoration process continued for many months.

Several years ago I started practicing yoga and found it a great tool for managing both stress and mood, while fine-tuning my body. Unfortunately, during the first four months after my disc ruptured, I couldn't go to yoga class because my back just wasn't ready for all the bending and twisting. This meant I couldn't utilize one of my biggest coping strategies, right when I needed it the most. Yet I knew it was important to "keep my head straight" so my mind could support my body's recovery, rather than work against it. So I consciously stopped myself from looking too far ahead and worrying about the future, and focused on the present. I routinely visualized success, imagining that my macrophages were chewing up extruded disc material every time I was on the acupuncture table. Breathing exercises and prayer were parts of my daily routine, and I tried to be grateful for each and every day, no matter how difficult it was. I felt fortunate that I could continue to work, especially since I'd seen so many patients lose their jobs, their homes, and their families due to back injuries.

Setting specific goals also proved helpful. I planned a hiking trip to Yosemite with my son during his spring break, and that gave me purpose: I really wanted to have that experience with him. In the months leading up to our trip, I gradually pushed my walking tolerance from a few blocks to a few miles, and went from walking on level ground to climbing up and down hills. Because my goal was so clear and so important to me, I made great strides in gaining endurance and strength. And I had a blast with my son.

My recovery process continues to unfold to this day. Even though I am still making progress, there have been a number of setbacks and bumps along the road. It seems that every time I take two steps forward, shortly thereafter something pushes me back a step. Conquering pain relief is a bumpy flight, with lots of turbulence. But in the long run, my results have been positive.

For any disease, injury, or other ailment of the flesh, there seems to be only two possible outcomes. You can get stuck in your pain and be unable to blossom, evolve, or find a more meaningful path forward. Or you can use adversity as an opportunity for growth, rejuvenation, and becoming stronger. In other words, you can turn your losses into gains. Doing this is one of life's greatest victories.

How sweet and beautiful is the spring that comes after the darkest of winters!

NOTES

Introduction

1. Gachel RJ, Okifuki A. Evidence-based scientific data documenting the treatment and cost-effectiveness of comprehensive pain programs for chronic nonmalignant pain. *J Pain*, 2006;7(11):779-93.

Chapter 2

1. "NIH-funded study suggests brain is hard-wired for chronic pain." National Institutes of Health, September 17, 2013. Accessible at *www.nih.gov/news/health/sep2013/ninds-17.htm*. Viewed August 4, 2014.

2. Mansour AR, Baliki MN, Huang L, Torbey S, et al. Brain white matter structural properties predict transition to chronic pain. *Pain*, 2013;154(10):2160-2168.

3. Baliki MN, Geha PY, Apkarian AV, Chialvo, DR. Beyond feeling: chronic pain hurts the brain, disrupting the default-mode network dynamics. *Journal of Neuroscience*, 2008:28(6):1398-1403.

4. Apkarian AV, Sosa Y, Krauss BR, Thomas PS, Fredrickson BE, Levy RE, Harden R, Chialvo DR. Chronic pain patients are impaired on an emotional decision-making task. *Pain*, 2004:108;129-136.

5. Study reveals brain mechanism behind chronic pain's sapping of motivation. Stanford Medicine News Center, July 31, 2014. Accessible at *http://med.stanford.edu/news/all-news/2014/07/study-reveals-brain-mechanism-behind-chronic-pains-sapping-of-mo.html*. Viewed August 4, 2014.

6. Chronic pain research delves into brain: New insight into how brain responds to pain. University of Adelaide, March 12, 2014. Accessible at

www.sciencedaily.com/releases/2014/03/140312103143.htm. Viewed August 4, 2014.

7.   Ji RR, Berta T, Nedergaard M. Glia and pain: is chronic pain a gliopathy? *Pain*, 2013;154 Suppl 1:S10-28.

8.   Mutso, A A, Radzicki D, Baliki M, et al. Abnormities in hippocampal functioning with persistent pain. *J Neuroscience*, 2012;32(17):5747-5756.

Chapter 3

1.   Meier, Barry. A soldier's war on pain. *New York Times*, May 10, 2014. Accessible at *www.nytimes.com/2014/05/11/business/a-soldiers -war-on-pain.html?_r=1*. Viewed September 11, 2014.

Chapter 5

1.   Martel MO, Wasan AD, Jamison RN, Edwards RR. Catastrophic thinking and increased risk for prescription opioid misuse in patients with chronic pain. *Drug and Alcohol Dependence*, 2013;132(1-2):335-41.

2.   Sullivan MJL, Lynch ME, Clark AJ. Dimensions of catastrophic thinking associated with pain experience and disability in patients with neuropathic pain conditions. *Pain*, 2005;113:310-315.

3.   Crombez G, Eccleston C, Van den Broeck A, Van Houdenhove B, Goubert L. The effects of catastrophic thinking about pain on attentional interference by pain; no mediation of negative affectively in healthy volunteers and in patients with low back pain. *Pain Research and Management*, 2002;7(1):31-9.

4.   Emmons, R. Gratitude works! The science and practice of saying thanks. YouTube. Accessible at *www.youtube.com/watch?v=BF7xS_nPbZ0*. Viewed August 10, 2015.

Chapter 6

1.   Boso M, et al. Neurophysiology and neurobiology of the musical experience. *Functional Neurology*, 2006;21(4):187-191.

Chapter 7

1.   Shnayderman, I, Katz-Leurer, M. An aerobic walking programme versus muscle strengthening programme for chronic low back pain: a randomized controlled trail. *Clinical Rehabilitation*, 2013;27:3207-214.

2.   Wells C, Kolt GS, Marshall P, et al. The effectiveness of Pilates exercise in people with chronic low back pain: a systematic review. *PLos ONE*, 9 (7):e100402. doi:10.1371/journal.pone.0100402.

3.   Yoga and stretching exercises beneficial for chronic low back pain, study finds. *Science Daily*, October 24, 2011. Accessible at *www .sciencedaily.com/releases/2011/10/111024164710.htm*. Viewed August 10, 2015.

4. Jones, KD, Adams D, Winters-Stone K, Burckhardt, CS. A comprehensive review of 46 exercise treatment studies in fibromyalgia (1988-2005). *Health and Quality of Life Outcomes*, 2006;4:67.

5. Splete, Heidi. Gentle yoga poses ease pain in women with fibromyalgia. *Clinical Psychiatry News*, December 2010:44.

6. Physical activity for arthritis fact sheet. Centers for Disease Control and Prevention. Last updated December 4, 2014. Accessible at *www.cdc .gov/arthritis/pa_factsheet.htm*. Viewed April 13, 2015.

7. Haaz, S, Bartlett SJ. Yoga for arthritis: a scoping review. *Rheumatic Disease Clinics of North America*, 2011;37(1):33-46.

8. White DK, Tudor-Locke C, Zhang Y, Fielding R, et al. Daily walking and the risk of incident functional imitation in knee osteoarthritis: an observational study. *Arthritis Care & Research*, 2014;66(9):1328-1336.

9. Kilgore WDS, Olson EA, Weber M. Physical exercise habits correlate with gray matter volume of the hippocampus in healthy adult humans. *Scientific Reports*, 2013;3:3457. Viewed April 13, 2015.

10. Erickson KI, Voss MW, Prakash RS, et al. Exercise training increases size of hippocampus and improves memory. *Proceedings of the National Academy of Sciences of the United States of America*, 2011;108(7):3017-3022.

11. Williamson, JW, Nobrega ACL, McColl R, et al. Activation of the insular cortex during dynamic exercise in humans. *Journal of Physiology*, 1997;503(2):277-283.

12. Tsujii T, Komatsu K, Sakatani K. Acute effects of physical exercise on prefrontal cortex activity in older adults: a functional near-infrared spectroscopy study. *Advances in Experimental Medicine and Biology*, 2013;765:293-298.

13. Greenwood BN, Foley TE, Le TV, Strong PV, et al. Long term voluntary wheel running is rewarding and produces plasticity in the mesolimbic reward system. *Behavioral Brain Research*, 2011;217(2):354-362.

14. Lehmann ML, Herkenham M. Environmental enrichment confers stress resiliency to social defeat through an infralimbic cortex-dependent neuroanatomical pathway. *Journal of Neuroscience*, 2011;31(16):6159-6173.

15. "Just 30 minutes of exercise has benefits for the brain." News & Events, The University of Adelaide. October 27, 2014. Accessible at *www .adelaide.edu.au/news/news74203.html*.

16. Schoenfeld, TJ, Rada P, Pieruzzini, Hsueh B, Gould E. Physical exercise prevents stress-induced activation of granule neurons and enhances local inhibitory mechanisms in the dentate gyrus. *Journal of Neuroscience*, 2013;33(18):7770-777.

17. Blumenthal, JA, Smith PJ, Hoffman, BM. Is exercise a viable treatment for depression? *American College of Sports Medicine's Health and Fitness Journal*, 2012;16(4):14-21.

Chapter 8

1. Cryan, JF, Dinan, TG. Mind-altering microorganisms: the impact of the gut microbiota on brain and behavior. *Nature Reviews Neuroscience*, 2012;13:701-712.
2. Mayer, EA. Gut feelings: the emerging biology of gut–brain communication. *Nature Reviews Neuroscience*, 2011;12:453–466.
3. Thaler JP, Yi CX, Schur EA, Guyenet SJ, Hwang BH, Dietrich MO. Obesity is associated with hypothalamic injury in rodents and humans. *Journal of Clinical Investigation*, 2012;122(1):153–162.

Chapter 9

1. Sivertsen B, Lallukka T, Petrie K, et al. Sleep and pain sensitivity in adults. *Pain*, 2015;1. doi:10.1097/j.pain.0000000000000131.
2. Griffin RM. 9 surprising reasons to get more sleep. WebMD. Page last reviewed December 27, 2011. Accessible at *www.webmd.com/sleep -disorders/features/9-reasons-to-sleep-more?page=3*. Page viewed April 15, 2015.
3. Roehrs, TA, Harris E, Randall S, Roth T. Pain sensitivity and recovery from mild chronic sleep loss. *Sleep*, 2012;35(12):1667-1672.
4. Chang PP, Ford DE, Mead LA, et al. Insomnia in young men and subsequent depression. The Johns Hopkins Precursors Study. *American Journal of Epidemiology*, 1997;146(2):105-114.
5. Dang-Vu TT, Desseilles M, Peigneux P, Maquet P. A role for sleep in brain plasticity. *Pediatric Rehabilitation*, 2006;9(2):92-118.
6. Kripke DF, Langer RD, Kline LE. Hypnotics' association with mortality or cancer: a matched cohort study. *British Medical Journal Open*, 2012;2:e000850. doi:10.1136/bmjopen-2012-000850
7. Morin CM, Vallieres A, Guay B, Ivers H, et al. Cognitive-behavioral therapy, singly and combined with medication, for persistent insomnia: acute and maintenance therapeutic effects. *Journal of the American Medical Association*, 2009;301(19):2005-2015.
8. Mitchel MD, Gehrman P, Perlis M, Umscheid CA. Comparative effectiveness of cognitive behavioral therapy for insomnia: a systematic review. *BMC Family Practice*, 2012;13:40.

INDEX

Abaci plan, 51-59
acceptance, 93-94
active body, 113-114, 117-118
active meditation, 71, 74-75
acupuncture, 137, 182
acute pain, 37-38, 118,
    131-132
Affordable Care Act
    (Obama Care), 32-33
alpha-lipoic acid, 142
American sleep cycles,
    149-150
amygdala, 46-48, 62, 66-67,
    84, 100, 106, 117
anger, 46-47, 56-57, 66, 69,
    71-72, 78, 84, 89-91, 94,
    97-98
anterior cingulate cortex
    (ACC), 47, 66-67, 115
anxiety, 21-22, 25, 39, 43, 46,
    53, 55, 64, 72, 77-78, 81,
    88, 94, 97, 106-107,
    117-118, 124-125, 129,
    131, 133, 136, 146
art therapy, 16, 71, 76-80,
    107-109, 160, 164
biopsychosocial model,
    13-14

brain blood flow, 42
breathing exercises, 27, 56, 71,
    75-77, 120, 152, 182
Bridge, The (art therapy exercise),
    78-79
buprenorphine, 137
catastrophic thinking, 56, 84-88,
    94, 97
central sensitization, 48, 56, 68
cognitive-behavioral therapy
    (CBT), 153-154
communicating with your doctor,
    161-163
compassion, 33, 56, 84, 95-97, 175
core strength, 121-122
cortisol, 47, 66-67, 107
creativity, 57, 99-110
crocheting, 109-110
daily gratitude, 94-95
dance therapy, 104-106, 156
depression, 15, 21-22, 25, 27-28,
    39, 43, 46, 49, 51, 53, 55, 66,
    71-72, 78, 88-89, 94, 97,
    104-106, 115, 118, 129, 131,
    133, 138, 147
diaphragmatic breathing, 76, 91
diffusion tensor imaging
    (DTI), 42

endocrine system, 65
essential fatty acids, 134
exercise, 111-126
eye movement desensitization
and reprocessing (EMDR), 56,
71, 81-82, 164
fatigue, 115, 129, 145, 147
fear avoidance, 118-119
fear, 22, 39, 46-47, 56-57, 66-67,
71, 73, 78, 84, 86, 88-89,
94, 98, 118-121, 124
fibromyalgia, 38, 114-115,
125, 131
fight or flight response, 47, 55,
63-66, 68-70, 73, 76, 87
finding calm in the storm, 55,
61-82, 1-7
fish oil, 142
4-7-8 breathing, 76-77
functional magnetic resonance
imaging (fMRI), 42
"fuzzy thinking," 43
gaining treatment perspective,
58, 155-165
glial cells, 41, 45-46, 129-130,
132-135, 138
glycemic load, 134-135
gray matter, 40-41, 101, 115,
125, 138
gut bacteria, 127-129
gut microbiome, 127-130,
132-133
health insurance companies, 14,
16-17, 26-28, 30-33, 38, 58,
89, 156-157, 164-165,
healthy brain, 22, 35, 43, 62, 66,
69, 115, 174
hippocampus, 47-48, 62, 67,
106, 115-116, 118, 133, 148
hypothalamus-pituitary-
adrenal axis, 47

independence, 54, 114, 161, 168
inflammation, 46, 58, 72, 97,
129-130, 133-135, 138-140,
142, 165
"ingesting quality," 58, 127-143
insomnia, 31, 146-148, 152-154
insula (insular cortex), 48, 62,
67, 115-116
interaction (social), 46-47, 53,
116, 160, 168, 170-171
knitting, 109-110
learned helplessness, 91-93,
learning, slowed, 44
love, 54, 56, 96-97, 161, 168, 170
magnetic resonance imaging
(MRI), 21, 29, 42, 54, 85, 165
mandala (art therapy exercise),
7-80
Mask, The (art therapy
exercise), 78
medical devices, 21, 32-33,
48, 163
medical studies, 159-161
Medicare, 27, 30, 165
Mediterranean diet, 138-140
mobility, 53, 141, 161, 168
motivation centers of the brain,
43-44
movement, 114-126
musculoskeletal problems,
122-123
music therapy, 106-107
myelinated nerve axons, 41
neurogenesis, 39-40
neurons, 39-41, 45-46, 133
neuroplasticity, 40, 44, 148
obesity, 128-130, 133, 135-136
opioids, 24-25, 31, 58, 86, 130-
133, 136-137
osteoarthritis, 115
pacing, 123-124

"pain body," 112-114 118-124, 135-136, 168, 177

"pain brain," 22, 27, 35, 37-48, 57-59, 70-71, 81, 100-103, 112-113, 115, 130, 132-133, 135-136, 164, 168-169, healing the, 53-55 stressed out, 66-68 therapeutic creativity and the, 100-101

pain equation, 49, 53, 84-85, 90, 94, 112-113, 117, 135, 146

pain-changed brain, 39-49

painkillers, 16, 25, 28, 51, 93, 147

pain-relief nutritional plan, 137-138

pain-relief village, 170-171

parasympathetic nervous system (PNS), 65-66, 80, 125

Pilates, 58, 114, 121-122, 125, 164

posttraumatic stress disorder (PTSD), 56

prefrontal cortex, 45-48, 84, 101, 116-117

pressure to prescribe medicines, doctors', 28-30

psoriatic arthritis, 128

qi gong, 114, 125

quilting, 109-110

recharging (sleeping), 58, 145-154

reframing harmful thoughts, 56, 86-87, 156

resiliency, 91-93, 94, 181

rheumatoid arthritis, 22, 38, 115, 128-130, 133, 138

self-efficacy, 174-176

sleep hygiene, 150-152

sleeping pills, 31, 58, 148-149, 152-154

somatosensory cortex, 45, 115

sorting through medical advice, 157-159

still meditation, 71-73

strength training, 114

stress, 45, 47-48, 62-63, 66-73, 75, 77, 80-81, 87, 90, 92, 94, 97, 101, 107, 110, 115, 117-118, 124-125, 128-130, 132, 135, 151, 171, 174

sun and moon breathing, 77

supplements, 127, 142-143

sympathetic nervous system (SNS), 65-66

tai chi, 58, 124-125, 164, 170

telling your story, 102-103

therapeutic creativity, 100-101

time (as a factor in healing), 168-170

time pressures, doctors', 27-28

trauma reactivation, 69-70

trauma, 68-69 chronic pain as a source of, 70

validation, 54, 161, 168, 170

vitamin D, 142-143

walking, 53, 57, 74-75, 114-116, 119, 125, 167, 170, 175

weight management, 135, 140-142

white matter "pain pattern," 41-42

workstation tips, 172-173

yoga, 56, 58, 71, 80-81, 114-115, 121-122, 125, 153

ABOUT THE AUTHOR

Peter Abaci, MD, is one of the world's leading experts on pain. He is the author of *Take Charge of Your Chronic Pain,* host of Health Revolution Radio, and a regular contributor to WebMD, *The Huffington Post,* and PainReliefRevolution.com. As the medical director and co-founder of the renowned Bay Area Pain & Wellness Center, his innovative strategies for integrative pain treatment have helped restore the lives of thousands struggling with pain. Dr. Abaci's publications on pain treatment have become a trusted resource for patients, family members, doctors, psychologists, physical therapists, and insurance companies alike. He resides with his family in Los Gatos, California. For more information, visit *www.peterabaci.com.*